OXFORD PSYCHOLOGY SERIES NO. 12

BLINDSIGHT

A Case Study and Implications

L. Weiskrantz
Professor of Psychology
University of Oxford

CLARENDON PRESS · OXFORD

Oxford University Press, Walton Street, Oxford OX2 6DP
Oxford New York Toronto
Delhi Bombay Calcutta Madras Karachi
Petaling Jaya Singapore Hong Kong Tokyo
Nairobi Dar es Salaam Cape Town
Melbourne Auckland
and associated companies in
Berlin Ibadan

Oxford is a trade mark of Oxford University Press

Published in the United States
by Oxford University Press, New York

British Library Cataloguing in Publication Data
Weiskrantz, Lawrence
Blindsight: a case study and implictions.
—(Oxford psychology series; 12)
1. Blind   2. Visual perception
I. Title
152.1'4   BF241
ISBN 0–19–852129–4
ISBN 0–19–852192–8 (Pbk)

Library of Congress Cataloging in Publication Data
Weiskrantz, Lawrence.
Blindsight: a case study and implications.
(Oxford psychology series; no. 12)
Bibliography: p.
Includes indexes.
1. Blindness—Case studies.   2. Visual cortex—
Diseases—Case studies.   3. Neuropsychology—Case
studies   I. Title. II. Series.
RE725.W45 1986   617.7   86-12515
ISBN 0–19–852129–4
ISBN 0–19–852192–8 (Pbk)

Typeset by Dobbie Typesetting Service, Plymouth, Devon
Printed in Great Britain by
J. W. Arrowsmith Ltd, Bristol

BLINDSIGHT

A Case Study and Implications

OXFORD PSYCHOLOGY SERIES

EDITORS
DONALD E. BROADBENT
JAMES L. MCGAUGH
NICHOLAS J. MACKINTOSH
MICHAEL I. POSNER
ENDEL TULVING
LAWRENCE WEISKRANTZ

Preface

The case study that forms a large part of this monograph was prompted by the astute observations of a clinical ophthalmic surgeon, Mr Michael Sanders, at the National Hospital, Queen Square, London, who first noticed unexpected signs of residual capacity within the 'blind' visual field of D.B., and reported his observations to Dr (now Professor) Elizabeth Warrington, of the same hospital. She, in turn, drew my attention to them, and together with Mr Sanders and Professor Marshall (in whose charge D.B. was a patient at the hospital) we published our first investigations in 1974, soon after the seminal report of Ernst Pöppel and his colleagues. Almost incidentally, we invented the term 'blindsight'. The name caught on, and unwittingly became attached not only to findings with D.B. but also, in other groups' studies, to a variety of aspects of residual vision in 'blind' fields caused by cortical brain damage, especially when there is a corresponding lack of awareness of the visual capacity by the patient. Perhaps the name has also contributed to the ease of reference and debate by experimental psychologists, neuroscientists, and philosophers of mind. Meanwhile, our research with D.B. continued for several years but much of it has remained unpublished until now. The time seems ripe, perhaps, to draw our corpus of findings together in one place, and to attempt to set them and the issues that emerge from them in the perspective of neurological findings and of other contemporary work.

Throughout the entire series of experimental studies reported here, spread over more than ten years, Elizabeth Warrington was a constant research collaborator. She shared in formulating the questions, designing the experiments, collecting every data point, proposing and discussing hypotheses. I had hoped that she would be a co-author of the whole, or failing that even a part, of this monograph, but she preferred the journal mode, especially as the review and interpretation sections of this monograph continuously expanded as they emanated from my word processor. I can only record my deepest appreciation and my debt of gratitude to her.

The National Hosital also provided testing space and help of various kinds over several years, for which I am very appreciative. The special and rare atmosphere at Queen Square in fostering neurological research helped to make such a study feasible. I am also grateful to technical staff in my own Department of Experimental Psychology at Òxford for much help with the peculiar demands I frequently put them for apparatus and photographic material, especially when we tested in Oxford. In particular, I thank Brian Baker, Roger Barnes, Ray Bennett, and Jeremy Broad.

I also acknowledge a special debt to the Medical Research Council, which supported my clinical research as part of a larger programme grant to Professor Alan Cowey and me. By very generously offering to take over my personal support completely from 1977 to 1979, the Council enabled me to put aside the demands of University administration and to devote myself fully to research. While it would have been an untold luxury to have had longer, I am grateful that Oxford University allowed me to stand down from my other duties during that period.

Oxford colleagues have provided much valuable discussion and criticism over several years. Among these, Alan Cowey, whose own scientific contribution to related aspects of this research will be evident to the reader, deserves special thanks. Parts of the material reviewed here have been published elsewhere in journals, and acknowledgements will be found in the text. I am very grateful to the Royal Society of London for making available the portrait of Gordon Holmes, which originally appeared in *Biographical Memoirs of Fellows of the Royal Society*, vol. 12 (1966).

Oxford University Press have been extraordinarily helpful and efficient at all stages of the publishing process, and it is a pleasure to express my thanks to them. I am also grateful to my wife for preparation of the indexes and help with the proofs.

Finally, of course, D.B. himself: a painstaking, forebearing, extremely cooperative and astute participant, observer, and commentator over so many days and days — and still more days — of testing, much of it no doubt very tedious to him. To him is owed an inestimable debt.

Oxford   L.W.
March 1986

Contents

Part I

1 Background

There is a paradox concerning the visual pathways and their functions. In man and other primates most of the fibres from the optic nerve leaving the eye project more or less directly to a region of the cerebral cortex situated at the most posterior region of the brain (Figs. 1 and 2), in a region known as the occipital lobe. The specific cortex within the occipital lobe which receives this visual input is called the 'striate cortex' because of its distinctive appearance under the microscope (also known as area 17, area OC, or V–1). Actually, the projection from eye to cortex is not absolutely direct: the optic nerve fibres themselves terminate in a nucleus of the thalamus in the 'tween-brain' (the diencephalon), in the dorsal lateral geniculate nucleus, and from that nucleus new fibres originate that terminate in the striate cortex. Hence,

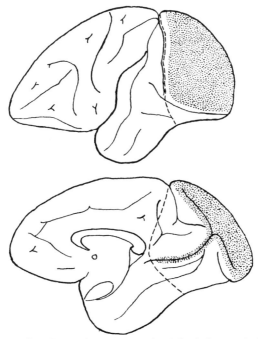

Fig. 1.   Lateral and medial views of monkey brain. Stippled areas indicate striate cortex. Dotted line indicates anterior limit of lesion if all striate cortex were to be removed by lobectomy method. Based on Brodman (1909), as redrawn by Marquis and Hilgard (1937). (Reprinted from Weiskrantz 1972, by permission)

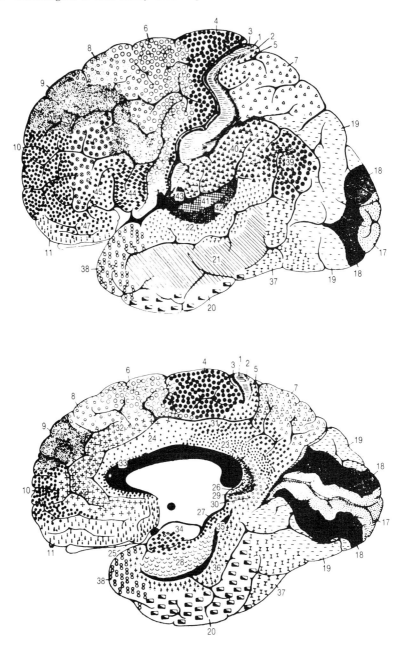

Fig. 2. Classification of human cortex by cytoarchetectonic criteria. Note that striate cortex (area 17) is largely buried in the calcarine fissure on the medial surface of the brain, and is complete surrounded by areas 18 and 19. (From Brodmann 1909, reprinted from Weiskrantz 1972, by permission)

this system is commonly designated as the 'geniculo-striate' pathway. But functionally speaking, the output from the eye has a relatively direct and strong impact upon the activity of the striate cortex. In fact, this anatomical projection is stronger than any other in the brain—about half of all the inputs into the brain are from fibres from the eye that have relatively direct and concentrated access to the cerebral cortex.

The paradox is this: while the geniculo-striate pathway constitutes the major portion of the optic nerve (containing about 90 per cent of its fibres), there are nevertheless several other branches of the optic nerve that take a different route. In fact, there are at least 6 other branches that end up in the midbrain and sub-cortical regions (Weiskrantz 1972), and one of these contains about 100 000 fibres, by no means a trivial pathway—it is larger than the whole of the auditory nerve (Fig. 3). Recently a projection (via a lateral geniculate relay) has also been discovered to *non*-striate cortex in the monkey (Yoshida and Benevento 1981; Fries 1981). Therefore, if striate cortex is removed or its direct input blockaded, one should expect that some visual capacity should remain because all of these non-geniculo-striate pathways are left intact. The paradox is that in man this is usually not so: destruction of occipital cortex— through strokes, tumours, disease, or accident—characteristically causes blindness in that part of the visual field corresponding to the precise projection map of the retina on to the striate cortex (Fig. 4). Admittedly, some primitive visual reflexes can be detected—the pupils still expand in darkness and

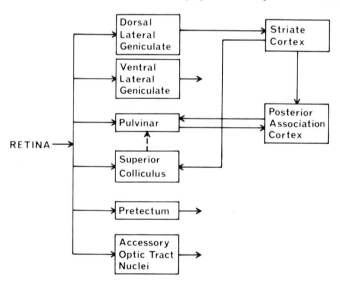

Fig. 3. A schema of some of the known outputs from the monkey retina. In addition to these pathways, there is now known to be a pathway from dorsal lateral geniculate nucleus to pre-striate cortex (posterior association cortex), and it is likely that a pathway exists from the retina to supra-chiasmatic nucleus of the hypothalamus— see text. (From Weiskrantz 1972, reprinted by permission)

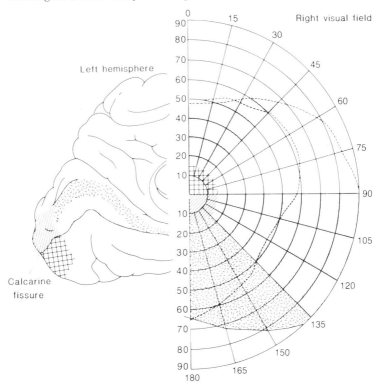

Fig. 4. Map of projection of the contralateral visual half-field on to striate cortex on the medial surface of the human brain. (From *Fundamentals of human neuropsychology*, by B. Kolb and I. Q. Whishaw. W. H. Freeman and Company. Copyright © 1985; adapted from Poggio (1968).)

contract in bright light, there *may* be opto-kinetic reflexes elicited by certain patterns of moving stimuli — but typically the patient himself does not appear to discriminate visual events or to have any awareness of them. From time to time there have been reports of exceptions to this generalization, made difficult to interpret because of the absence of precise knowledge of the locus of the brain damage (Weiskrantz 1961), but William James's conclusion of almost 100 years ago is still apt as a summary of present-day clinical wisdom: 'The literature is tedious *ad libitum*. . . . The occipital lobes are indispensable for vision in man. Hemiopic disturbance comes from lesion of either one of them, and total blindness, sensorial as well as psychic, from destruction of both.' (James 1890, p. 47). The disturbance is hemiopic, i.e., affecting only a half-field of vision, because each occipital lobe receives an input from the half of *both* retinae from the same side of the body: the left half of each retina projects to the left occipital lobe and the right half of each retina to the right. Because the visual image is inverted on the retina, the result is that the right half of the field of vision is affected by left hemisphere lesions, and the left field of vision by right hemisphere lesions — see below.

If it were the case that the animal evidence also agreed with that from the human clinic, the paradox might simply boil down to the conclusion that the extra-striate pathways mediated primitive reflexes and nothing else, even though more than 100 000 fibres seems rather an excessive ration for such a role. But the paradox has been made larger, not smaller, as animal evidence has accumulated. Even in William James's time, there was evidence that removal of the occipital lobes in monkeys did not cause absolute blindness (although James himself misquotes the available evidence from Munk that it did, cf. Weiskrantz 1980). Munk and Schäfer both agreed that 'after a certain time vision partially returns.' More surprisingly, perhaps, Ferrier had earlier argued that there was no effect whatever on vision: 'I removed the greater portion of both occipital lobes at the same time without causing the slightest appreciable impairment of vision. One of these animals within two hours of the operation was able to run about freely, avoiding obstacles, to pick up such a minute object as a raisin without the slightest hesitation or want of precision, and to act in accordance with its visual experience in a perfectly normal manner.' (Ferrier, 1886). Ferrier became locked in a bitter dispute with Schäfer over such an extreme claim, and with benefit of hindsight it appears likely that Ferrier's lesions were incomplete — but at that time precise anatomical information about the visual pathways was incomplete. James himself sided with Munk, but hedged: he said the procedure 'makes the animal *almost* blind.' But 'as for the crude sensitivity to light which *may* then remain, nothing exact is known either about its nature or its seat.' (James 1890, p. 63, italics added).

That monkeys without striate cortex *could* respond to light was established firmly in the first half of the present century, which could also benefit from more solid anatomical knowledge. Thus, Marquis and Hilgard (1937) showed that the conditioned eyelid response to light (with air puff as the unconditioned stimulus) could be demonstrated in monkeys with complete removal of striate cortex (and with confirmed complete degeneration of the lateral geniculate nucleus). They also noted head turning and reaching toward visual objects or shadows, but they were cautious in drawing any conclusions because of the possibility of auditory cues). But the work that first dealt with the question at the animal level in more systematic and quantitative terms was that of Klüver (1942). Using formal tests of visual discrimination in which monkeys were trained to respond to particular stimuli to obtain food reward, he concluded that in the absence of striate cortex monkeys could react only to the total amount of luminous energy and not to the pattern of its distribution. For example, a large dim square would be treated as the same as a small bright square if both reflected or transmitted equal amounts of total light energy. The animal behaved, as it were, as a photo-cell does — sensitive to light stimulation, but not to the shape or arrangement of the stimulation.

The matter rested there for more than two decades, but subsequent work has shown that Klüver's results and characterization were far too limited. One of the clues came from an observation that emerged almost by chance due to a practical difficulty in obtaining, in the time available, varying shades of grey paper which were intended to be used to match the flux of a striped grating—it being predicted that a monkey without striate cortex would find the task impossible to discriminate between the two. For practical reasons, an attempt was made to simulate grey by cutting up black and white segments into small pieces which produced a kind of very fine 'salt and pepper' arrangement. Surprisingly the animal found it relatively easy to discriminate this salt and pepper field from black and white stripes exactly matched in total luminous flux (Weiskrantz 1963; cf. also account by Teuber 1965). On this basis, it was suggested that Klüver's characterization could be extended to include not only total amount of light energy associated with a visual stimulus, but also total amount of contour information, or 'edginess'. As it happened the initial unexpected results required further replication, which was duly achieved, because subsequent histology of this first animal's brain revealed a small number of intact cells in the lateral geniculate nucleus (which undergoes retrograde degeneration after striate cortex removal: the small cluster of cells indicated that there must have been a small amount of striate cortex left intact corresponding to a far peripheral part of the visual field).

But by the time the replication had been carried out it was already clear that the expanded interpretation did not go nearly far enough. Noticing, as Denny-Brown and Chambers had done earlier (1955), that a monkey with a bilateral striate cortex lesion would appear to respond to moving stimuli and to follow them with eye movements, Humphrey taught animals to respond to a variety of 'salient' visual events with a technique of elegant simplicity. He required an animal merely to reach out and touch the source of a visual event to obtain food reward. Having done this, he then systematically varied the properties of the visual stimuli. He found that a monkey with a bilateral occipital lesion was exquisitely sensitive to small objects and to their spatial location in a way that Klüver could not have predicted (Humphrey 1970; Humphrey and Weiskrantz 1967). Following on from that, Weiskrantz, Cowey, and Passingham (1977) showed that after striate cortex removal monkeys can locate stimuli randomly located in space—not quite as accurately as they could preoperatively, but nevertheless very well—and do this even with durations too brief to allow an eye movement to be executed before the stimulus disappeared.

Pedro and Tauba Pasik and their colleagues have demonstrated that a monkey with complete removal of striate cortex can learn a pattern discrimination and also a brightness discrimination, both with total flux of the stimuli equated (Pasik and Pasik 1971; Schilder, Pasik, and Pasik 1971, 1972). In doing so, they have emphasized the crucial importance of the details of the training methods. They have also provided details of the fineness of discrimination of which such monkeys are capable. The animals have a reduced acuity and also require greater contrast to detect gratings, but nevertheless they are able to detect gratings of up to 11 cycles/degree, which means that they can detect a separation of about 2¾ minutes of arc between lines in the grating (Miller, Pasik, and Pasik 1980). They are also able to discriminate between lines in which the only difference is their orientation: they can discriminate a difference in orientation of about 8°, which is a good (although reduced) capacity level (Pasik and Pasik 1980).

And so Klüver's characterization will not hold: monkeys lacking striate cortex can detect stimuli of brief duration, and can locate them in space. They can detect the fine spatial separation between lines in a grating. They can discriminate differences of orientation in the frontal plane, and they can carry out simple form discriminations. There is also one claim that they have some residual colour vision (Schilder *et al.* 1972), although this requires further exploration given Humphrey's negative results (1970). None of these capacities would be possessed by a photo-cell type of capacity that integrated all sources of stimulation across the cell. Admittedly, some special controls would be needed to rule out the possibility that some of the discriminations might be based on scanning or other eye movement stratagems, much as a photo-cell at the end of a moving stalk might deliver different outputs to different stimuli. But such an explanation can be ruled out when the stimuli are brief, as was the case with the spatial location study of Weiskrantz *et al.* (1977).

The explanation of why Klüver obtained a much more limited capacity now seems clear. Unfortunately, histological reconstructions of the Klüver's lesions were never published, but fortunately the brains were preserved. The Pasiks have been able to examine them and they describe the lesions as including the whole of the striate cortex, but *also* involving additional cortex lying anterior to it and extending down into the temporal lobes. When they replicated Klüver's surgery, they also confirmed his behavioural findings as regards total luminous flux. In contrast, however, when the lesions were less extensive but nevertheless included all of the striate cortex — histologically confirmed by uniform degeneration of cells throughout the whole lateral geniculate nucleus — they found the much greater residual capacity, both quantitatively and qualitatively, just described above.

So far we have considered only the paradox that arises out of studies in which the geniculo-striate system has been completely bypassed by total removal of the striate cortex. But in the clinic it is extremely rare to find a patient with bilateral damage such that both half-fields are affected over their full extent. Much more commonly, patients have unilateral damage of varying extents and severity, leading to a local region of blindness — a 'scotoma'. When the lesion includes the whole of the striate cortex in the contralateral hemisphere, the entire half-field is affected, producing a 'hemianopia'. Because the patient is able to use the intact regions of his visual fields, he is not nearly so impaired in his everyday life as when the blindness covers the whole field, but within the scotoma the blindness is nevertheless severe. This is studied by using a 'perimeter' or a screen which allows one to present stimuli of controlled and specified dimensions in any region of the visual field.

Studies of animals with lesions of just part of the striate cortex do nothing to diminish the discrepancy between human clinical observations and animal evidence of residual visual function. On the contrary, if anything the discrepancy is more striking. It is the case that, as in man, restricted lesions within one hemisphere produce local impairments in vision approximately where they would be predicted from known anatomy and electrophysiology. But from the studies of Cowey (1963; cf. also Cowey and Weiskrantz 1963; Weiskrantz and Cowey 1970), several important qualifications must be made: First, the visual defect is by no means an absolute one; the intensity has to be reduced very substantially below the training level before the scotoma can be defined reliably. Second, the ability of the monkey to detect a given stimulus intensity within the scotoma improves markedly and radically over several months of postoperative testing. If the intensity is not reduced in order to compensate for this improvement, it may be impossible to reveal any detection impairment at all. Third, there is a gradual shrinkage of the *size* of the defective region of vision. Fourth, the impairment is not uniformly distributed, but is highest in the centre of the defective region and lowest at the edges. Fifth, the gradual improvement in visual sensitivity appears not to occur spontaneously, but requires very specific training directed towards requiring the animal to use its defective region. In fact, this requirement can be astonishingly specific. Mohler and Wurtz (1977) have shown that if an animal is given training to respond to brief and small flashes of light in only one *part* of the scotoma, that part recovers more than the remainder of the scotoma. It must be borne in mind that the whole of the scotoma is inevitably always being stimulated in the animal's normal waking hours, and so it is not stimulation *per se* that is important for recovery: it is the requirement that the animal actually respond to stimulation within the defective region, to make use of it.

The capacity of the defective region can be studied by measuring not only its sensitivity to the intensity of light, but also its resolving power or acuity. This is done by training the animal to respond to a fine grating in which the spacing and thickness of the lines can be varied. As the lines become narrower and more closely packed, a point is reached where they can no longer be distinguished from a homogeneous field (matched in luminous flux). The use of an acuity measure has a special advantage because it is well known that the grain, or 'packing' of the receptors on the retina is not uniform, and that acuity falls off sharply away from the fovea, the point on the retina which is the 'fixation point'. The monkey's acuity after a small central scotoma has been induced (by making a small bilateral striate cortex lesion) is reduced less than would be predicted by the electrophysiological maps of the visual fields onto striate cortex (Weiskrantz and Cowey 1963, 1967). When a scotoma is induced by small retinal lesions, in contrast, the reduction follows the prediction closely.

Given all this evidence of residual capacity within a scotoma affecting only part of the visual field, which pathways are responsible? Of course, as part of the visual field is intact, one must take special pains to rule out a false result that might stem from the use of the intact field. For example, there might be diffusion of light within the eye so that some of it spreads into the intact field and provides a kind of subtle cue about the presence of a visual event. Or the eyes may move rapidly to bring a stimulus into the intact field. Control experiments discount such false conclusions. For example, if the scotoma is caused by a small retinal lesion rather than a striate cortex lesion, then no recovery takes place nor is there any shrinkage of the field defect, despite the use of the same methods of testing as after striate cortex lesions. Brief stimuli make explanations in terms of a rapid switch of eye position quite impossible because they can be made to disappear before the eye has any chance to move to 'capture' them. There is, also, within each eye a built-in device that allows one to set very strict limits on the spread of light: the 'natural blind-spot', approximately 5° by 7° just where the optic nerve penetrates the retina and where, therefore, there are no light receptors. If one can plot this blind-spot in the animal with one's range of stimuli, it follows that the light could not have diffused in a useful way more than 2.5° (half the smaller dimension) in the eye, and probably much less than that. This is a trivial amount in relation to the size of residual visual phenomena. Finally, with the measurement of visual acuity, not only do the retinal lesion controls behave differently, but in fact diffusion of light within the eye would so seriously degrade the sharpness needed for visual discrimination that it could not be a viable explanation (Weiskrantz 1972, 1980).

When the lesion only includes part of the striate cortex in one hemisphere, there is a logical possibility that not only non-geniculo-striate pathways but also the intact striate cortex may play a role in allowing residual vision to occur. Intact striate cortex seems a reasonable possibility to account for the better than predicted visual acuity (Weiskrantz 1972). As regards the recovery of sensitivity to detect a brief and small flash of light, however, there is good evidence that a midbrain pathway accounts for the recovery. Mohler and Wurtz (1977) carried out an experiment in three stages. First, they made a small striate cortex lesion and plotted the scotoma that ensued. Next, they gave specific training in which the animal was rewarded for detecting stimuli within the scotoma, and as expected the scotoma gradually shrank and the animal's sensitivity returned. Finally, they made a small lesion in just that part of the superior colliculus, in the midbrain, to which the recovered part of the visual field is known to project. After the superior colliculus lesion, the scotoma was promptly reinstated and remained permanently, even with further training. Interestingly, in another experiment by these workers it was found that a superior colliculus lesion alone — without the antecedent striate cortex lesion — did not cause a scotoma, and so the conclusion must be that the superior colliculus came into play after the striate cortex lesion in such a way as to aid performance in this particular context.

And so, as animal evidence has progressed, there has been increasing evidence, with either partial or total lesions of the striate cortex, of residual visual function that has served to widen the gap between the results with human and subhuman subjects. With monkeys the paradox about a capacity of non-geniculo-striate pathways to mediate discriminative visual responses in the absence of the striate cortex has gradually dissolved. What has increasingly intruded is the paradoxical apparent difference between animals and man in this regard. The difference is probably not one simply of stimulus parameters used in testing, because Cowey and Weiskrantz (unpublished) have tested human patients in the same perimeter in which monkeys have been tested, and the scotomata in patients are far more severe than any seen in monkeys with striate cortex lesions. This difference was already a source of much interest and speculation 100 years ago; we have seen that William James was already aware of it.

One response has been to appeal to a doctrine of encephalization. Many reviewers (e.g., Monokow 1914; Marquis 1935) have attempted to arrange observations on subhuman animals in relation to human clinical observations into a phylogenetic series. The higher the phylogenetic status of the animal, it has been claimed, the more vision is dependent upon the visual cortex and its integrity. The view, in some ways, carries some curious implications (cf. Weiskrantz 1961, 1977). For example, is a midbrain pathway to the superior colliculus of some 100 000 fibres in the man merely vestigial? Another response has been to say that man is unique, and that anatomical similarity is not a reliable predictor of functional similarity. It would be desirable to try to resolve the discrepancy within a common neurological framework.

While reports of scotomata of absolute blindness caused by cerebral lesions are commonplace in the clinic, there are also scotomata of only relative blindness, i.e., of decreased sensitivity, and there have been some even more extreme claims. Many of these emerged from studies and surveys of soldiers who sustained gunshot head wounds in battle. Poppelreuter, who had extensive experience of First World War brain injury cases, declared that he could never find an *absolutely* blind scotoma; some rudimentary function was always present. He tried to order the different levels of visual function as follows: amorphous light sensitivity, size perception without definite form, amorphous form perception, perception of discrete objects, mild amblyopia, and normal vision (cited by Klüver 1927). Marie and Chatelin (1915) reported that in their examination of gunshot wound cases in the war they did not encounter anything but transient blindness, which was also the experience of Wilbrand and Saenger (1918). In such cases histological verification is rare, and it is difficult to separate the effects of shock, infection, vascular changes, and general dysfunction from more specific and enduring deficits.

In contrast stands the classical evidence of Gordon Holmes (Fig. 5) from the First World War. It was on the basis of careful and painstaking quantitative correlations between the details of the brain wounds and the scotomata that Holmes (1918) was able to construct the classical map of the visual fields upon the striate cortex (Fig. 6) that has stood the test of time and has been confirmed in its major features with the outcome of occipital damage due to a variety of causes. Holmes supported the view, at least in his early writings, that the resulting scotoma can be absolute and stable over long periods of time. He summarized the absolute character of the scotomata as follows: 'In all my cases [which appear black on the perimetry charts] the blindness was total to both white and colours; neither the presence nor the movement of any object or reasonable size could be recognized. It is, however, common to find a zone of indistinct or partial vision around the scotomata or on the borders of a quandrantic or incomplete hemianopia. . . . In the majority of my cases, however, which were examined more than three weeks after the onset of the blindness, the margins of the scotomata were

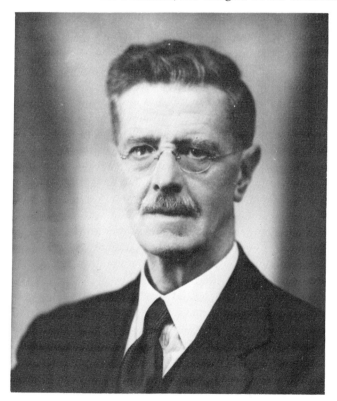

Fig. 5. Portrait of Gordon Holmes. (Courtesy of the Royal Society of London)

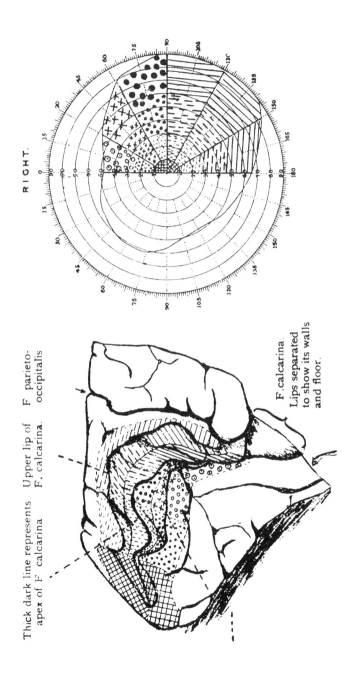

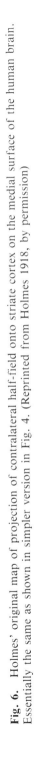

Fig. 6. Holmes' original map of projection of contralateral half-field onto striate cortex on the medial surface of the human brain. Essentially the same as shown in simpler version in Fig. 4. (Reprinted from Holmes 1918, by permission)

remarkably sharp; several patients, for instance, said when they first saw the object as it moved from the blind into the seeing area that "it seemed to come suddenly from behind a screen." ' (Holmes 1918, p. 378).

The analyses of gun-shot cases from the Second World War (Teuber, Battersby, and Bender 1960) also bore out Holmes's contention that scotomata could be absolutely blind, although they noted that under special conditions *some* of their cases showed some reactions to light in their seemingly blind scotomata, e.g., in responding to rapidly flickering stimuli or bright lights after dark adaptation. Because of the problem of diffusion of light into intact fields, however, they do not consider their evidence (nor Poppelreuter's) to be conclusive. It is of interest to note, however, that in his Ferrier Lecture some 27 years after his First World War survey Holmes had reached a more flexible position.

'The conclusions that can be drawn from observations on human subjects therefore indicate that in man primary visual perception . . . is subserved by the cortex of the striate area, and that though there is an exact geometric or point-to-point projection of the retina on this area its functional organization is not rigidly determined by this point-to-point representation, but is to some extent plastic or modifiable.'

(Holmes 1945, pp. 360–1).

There have been other reports that there may be some visual responsiveness in visual fields that are judged to be densely and absolutely blind in the perimeter: patients may respond to changes in intensity, movement, and flicker. For example, Bender and Krieger report that one of their patients was a man who

'had been completely blind for many years. When he was examined under ordinary room daylight, he could not tell whether it was light or dark. He was then placed in a dark room for 15 minutes, after which a brilliant light . . . was turned on and off. Precautions were taken to eliminate auditory and thermal cues. Nevertheless, the patient could tell the difference between light and dark.'

(Bender and Krieger 1951, p. 77).

More specific dissociations can also occur so that, for example, a patient may be able to respond well to moving stimuli but be blind for stationary stimuli (Riddoch 1917), and more surprisingly, just the complementary syndrome in which a subject is able to see a stationary object perfectly well but not when it is in movement (Zihl *et al.* 1983; cf. also Klüver 1927, for review of older clinical reports). There are, in fact, a whole range of other dissociable and occasionally relatively isolated visual disorders, e.g., of colour, spatial localization, but that interesting topic takes us beyond the immediate issue under review.

Perhaps the most conservative conclusion to draw from the clinical literature is that there are certainly some cases with field defects of absolute and permanent blindness, as assessed by a range of standard methods —

they are seen everyday by neurologists—and there are other cases in whom the defect is only relative and in whom there may also be recovery. There may be, as Holmes said, mixed cases in which an absolute scotoma is surrounded by one of only relative loss of sensitivity. But the clinical evidence suffers from two serious inadequacies. The first is that the methods of testing are often insensitive—for good reasons: clinical testing is designed for diagnostic purposes, not to advance an issue in research. Perimeters will show the shape of a defect, but without wide ranges of intensity and perhaps of duration of stimuli, will not show its precise size or its sensitivity. Research methods can be applied as research issues become sharpened, as in the suggestion of Teuber *et al.* (1960) that prolonged dark adaptation should be a feature of a search for residual light perception in a field defect. On the other hand, animal work has developed different and particular research methods that stem from particular questions, and also from the very special demands of animal testing itself.

But there is a second, much more intransigent issue, namely that in a human patient one rarely has adequate information on the precise site or limits of the lesion in the occipital lobe. This information, however, is of crucial importance. Let us remind ourselves of the apparent discrepancy between monkey and human results. In the monkey, if the lesion is restricted to the striate cortex the field defect is never absolute. If the lesion also includes additional cortex lying anterior to the striate cortex, residual vision is still present but is seriously degraded. In man, we sometimes have an absolute defect, and sometimes do not, after a lesion to the occipital lobe. But are those cases in which there is residual vision in man due, as Holmes argued, to an incomplete lesion of the striate cortex ('severe lesions of the visual cortex produce complete blindness . . . or if incomplete an amblyopia, colour vision being generally lost and white objects appearing indistinct, or only more potent stimuli, as abruptly moving objects, may excite sensations'. (1918, p. 384). Or is it that a field defect that is completely blind is caused by striate cortex damage *plus* additional damage, and that in man as in monkey if the damage were restricted to the striate cortex there would be a discriminative capacity that is greater than between mere changes in total light energy?

In fact, it turns out that the sheer geography of the human brain makes it extremely unlikely that a lesion would affect just striate cortex alone. In man the striate cortex lies almost entirely buried within a sulcus on the medial surface of the brain, whereas in the monkey much more is exposed on the lateral surface (Figs. 1 and 2). This means that in man it would be unusual for there to be a striate cortex lesion that did not also involve prestriate and other cortex, whereas in animal research a lesion restricted to striate cortex alone can be placed with some accuracy. The implication is, of course, that human defects may be more severe because the lesion would almost always include more than striate cortex alone. Cases of relatively restricted visual cortex damage in man, therefore, assume special importance, and it was observations on one such patient that led to the research reported in this monograph.

Thus far, our review of comparisons of field defects in man and monkey have been one of degree of severity, with the implication that the difference is quantitative only. It is as though the monkey's residual vision is somewhat like Holmes's description of an incomplete visual cortex in man, producing an amblyopia, i.e., indistinct, blurred and colour-free vision, what J. Loeb (1886) described in the dog without visual cortex as a 'dimness of vision', in which the affected part of the visual field suffers from an increased 'inertia' which can be partially overcome with 'stronger' or more 'salient' stimuli, as when a piece of food is moved in the impaired field. It is something like our looking at a scene with only our far peripheral vision. Indeed, at one time the monkey's residual vision was described in just this way (Weiskrantz 1972). But there are reasons for believing that the monkey, while it shows

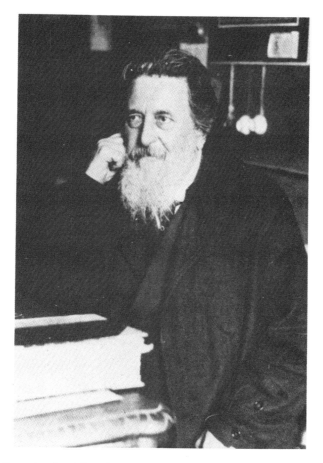

Fig. 7. Portrait of Luigi Luciani. (Reprinted by permission from Haymaker 1953.)

quite remarkable residual sensitivity to light and has other discriminative powers, is nevertheless altered in a *qualitative* way by striate cortex lesions. Perhaps the first investigator to have stressed this was the Italian physiologist, Luciani (Fig. 7). He asked: 'Are the visual *perceptions* . . . or are the simple *sensations* localized [in the visual cortical centres of the monkey]?' His answer was perfectly clear:

> 'When some time has elapsed after the extirpation, their visual sensation become perfect again; they are able to see minute objects, what they want is the discernment of things and a right judgement concerning their properties and their nature; they are deficient, in a word, of visual perception. For example, if small pieces of fig, mixed with pieces of sugar, are offered to them, they are incapable of choosing by sight alone but require to take the sugar in their hand and put it in their mouth in order to reassure themselves. . . . The animal is not able to distinguish meat from sugar by its visual impressions only.'
>
> (Luciani 1884, p. 153).

A highly similar conclusion was reached independently by Humphrey some 90 years later; he who studied a single monkey, Helen, over a period of several years in a variety of relatively naturalistic settings, and came to know her extremely well (Humphrey 1970, 1972, 1974). He demonstrated that she was exquisitely sensitive in locating and picking up small objects, such as tiny specks of paper, but she could not distinguish a bit of paper from a small peanut until she touched them, although she responded to either with fine sensitivity. She remained unable to identify even those things most familiar to her: 'After six years she still does not know a carrot when she sees one, nor apparently can she recognize my face, despite an excellent ability to locate visual events in her environment and to avoid obstacles by vision alone' (Humphrey 1972, p. 684). Cowey had earlier shown that a monkey after a unilateral striate cortex removal recovered much of its fine sensitivity to brief and small light stimuli in its hemianopic field. But when a strange doll was suspended in the 'monkey perimeter' to fall entirely within the impaired field, the animal continued to behave normally and ignored it altogether, although monkeys normally respond with some considerable vigour to strange dolls (Cowey 1961; Cowey and Weiskrantz 1963). When the same doll was suspended in the intact half-field, the animal reacted with cries of surprise and refused to test while the doll remained there.

This sort of observation suggests that what the monkey lacks is the ability to *identify* a visual object. He may be able to detect that something is present with fine sensitivity, and to locate it, but he requires striate cortex to know *what* it is. As such, the observations fit well into a general framework that emerged from a variety of sources that is commonly labelled as the 'two-visual systems' theory. In the strong form, the argument is that the midbrain pathways from the eye essentially mediate detection and localization of a visual event, and the striate cortex its identification (Ingle 1967; Schneider 1967; Trevarthen 1967). It is as though, to paraphrase William James, the main function of the midbrain system is that of 'sentinels which, when beams of light move over them, cry: "Who goes there?" ' and call the cortex to the spot. In detail the theory is not free from controversy, but it does serve to focus attention on distinct capacities for detection and localization that remain intact after interruption of the geniculo-striate system. It was this focus that led directly to a search for such a capacity in man.

The first positive clue came from a study by Pöppel, Held, and Frost in 1973. They were interested in whether stimuli projected into the field defects could exercise any control over eye movements. Animal evidence by Denny-Brown and Chambers (1955) and Humphrey (1970; Humphrey and Weiskrantz 1967) had both suggested that animals with bilateral striate cortex lesions would still direct their eyes to a novel visual event. Pöppel *et al.* flashed a light briefly in different locations of the field defects caused by gun-shot wounds in war veterans, and encouraged them to look in the direction in which the flash had occurred. This caused some considerable puzzlement in their subjects, because they could not actually 'see' the flash, but with encouragement they 'played the game' and looked in the direction where they somehow guessed the unseen flash had occurred. The eye movements were measured. There was a weak but positive correlation between the original target position and the position taken up by the eye, at least for eccentricities out to about 25°.

This observation was published soon before the time that the person of this monograph, D.B., came to our attention. There was, in a clinical setting, some independent indication that he could respond to the location of visual events in his blind hemianopic field (see below). D.B. attracted our attention for another reason: his defect was caused by the surgical removal of a small tumour of a blood vessel buried in the calcarine sulcus, which is where the striate cortex is located in man. Surgical notes were available that provided some of the dimensions of the likely lesion, and it seemed likely that it would be largely restricted to the striate cortex. Hence, he might provide more reasonable comparison with the results of animal studies and might help to resolve the discrepant findings. Finally, a study had just completed of the ability of monkeys to detect and locate visual events after striate cortex removal (although not actually published until a few years later, Weiskrantz *et al.* 1977) as an extension of a methodology earlier used by Humphrey. And so this provided an even greater opportunity to make a more direct comparison between man and monkey in which not only the lesion, but also the methodology was more closely equated. It was from such a background that D.B. offered to us this rare opportunity and privilege.

2 D.B.: Clinical history and early testing

D.B. was born in a small English market town in 1940. His childhood appears to have been uneventful medically, until the age of about 14 when he began to experience headaches. The headaches had a prelude: they were almost always preceded by a sensation of a flashing light, which appeared in an oval-shaped area immediately to the left of the centre of his visual field and straddling the horizontal axis. Then, over the course of a few minutes the oval enlarged, mainly in a downwards direction. After about 15 minutes the flashing lights in the oval stopped and the oval was blind. Its general appearance was of a white opaque area with a crescent of coloured lights around its outer and lower edges. This was the stage at which a headache would ensue, on the right side of his head. It was often followed by vomiting about 15 minutes later. The headache would persist for up to 48 hours, but usually he slept and upon waking would find his vision normal and his headache gone.

The attacks occurred at intervals of about six weeks until his twenties, when their frequency increased to one about every three weeks. Following one such attack he noticed he had a persistent field defect, smaller than the scotoma of his attacks. It appeared more as a blank than as a white oval, and was situated to the left of the fixation and more below than above the horizontal axis. He also occasionally had disturbances of touch down the left side of his body.

When he was 26 years old an angiogram was performed. This is a procedure in which a radio-opaque substance is injected into the blood stream and an X-ray picture taken of the head. Distortion in the position of cerebral blood vessels suggests a malformation in the brain. D.B.'s angiogram showed an arteriovenous malformation at the pole of the right occipital lobe. Such a malformation typically consist of a torturous mass of enlarged vessels of the cortex (Brain 1981, p. 243). It was hoped that drugs could control the migraine attacks, but these gave no relief. In 1970 relief of the pain was attempted by performing a surgical interruption of the sympathetic nervous system on the right side, in the region of the neck. The dilation of the cerebral arteries is influenced by the sympathetic nervous system, and it was thought that the dilation could be responsible for the migraine. Impulses giving rise to pain are transmitted by nerve fibres from the walls of the blood vessels. But this surgical treatment also provided no relief for D.B.

By now the attacks were causing a serious threat to D.B.'s family and social life, as well as to his employment, and in the absence of effective relief by any other treatment, in 1973 Professor Valentine Logue, at the National Hospital, Queen Square, London, surgically removed the malformation from the brain. From the surgical notes it was estimated that the excision extended from the occipital pole forward by approximately 6 cm and was thought to include the major portion of the calcarine cortex—in which the striate cortex is situated—on the medial surface of the right hemisphere. As can be seen from Holmes's classical drawing with a scale of the human brain (Figs 8 and 9), 6 cm is the approximate length of the calcarine fissure.

One effect of the operation was to cause the changes in his vision which are our main interest here. In terms of his general well-being, the surgery relieved his symptoms and indeed resulted in a positive transformation of

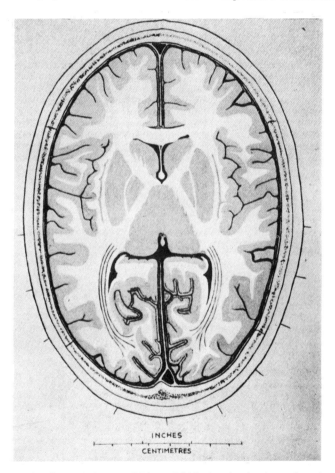

Fig. 8. Drawing from Holmes and Lister (1916) showing horizontal section through human brain at level of calcarine fissure. Location of striate cortex is shown by lightly dotted lines. (Reprinted by permission)

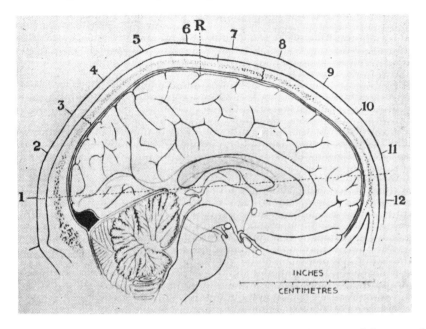

Fig. 9. Drawing from Holmes and Lister (1916) showing view of medial aspect of the human brain. (Reprinted by permission)

his day to day life. In the immediate post-operative period, for about five weeks, he reported seeing flashing lights in his left half-field, but these gradually subsided and then disappeared. They have been absent ever since, except for one episode (see below). He has remained largely free of headaches, although he does complain of the occasional migraine headache. His health has been excellent. He has been actively employed, and holds a responsible post in a small family business. His hobbies involve him in vigorous outdoor activities, such as scuba diving, and he is a keen musician in a local dance band. There is no doubt that the surgery transformed his state from one of severe handicap and painful discomfort to one that allows him to enjoy an active and enriching existence.

After operation most of D.B.'s left half-field was blind, as predicted. The hemianopia extended from the vertical meridian (there was no sparing of the macular field, as sometimes occurs in hemianopias; the macular field is a circular area of about 5°–10° surrounding the fixation point). The hemianopia was homonymous, i.e., it had the same shape and density in both eyes. By conventional perimetry, using the brightest and largest stimuli available (1° 40′ diameter, 1.2 log ft lamberts, 3 log units above background level), or using a brighter and larger display (see below), the defect was absolutely blind; he reported seeing nothing in his left half-field—except

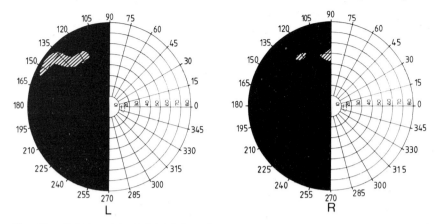

Fig. 10. D.B.'s original field defect eight months postoperatively, measured on a Goldmann perimeter, 1° target, maximum contrast. Hatched areas indicate amblyopic regions of preserved but hazy vision. (Redrawn from Weiskrantz *et al.* 1974, by permission)

however, in a crescent of preserved but fuzzy vision at the periphery of the upper quadrant (see Fig. 10).

His scotoma remained more or less constant in size, shape, and density until early in 1976, when he telephoned to say that he had had some return of vision in the upper part of the field defect. He was admitted to the National Hospital over the next two days for neurological examinations (which were unremarkable), and for the administration of further visual tests. In describing the return of function, D.B. reported that he experienced intermittent and small flashing lights near the region that remained blind.

Visual field plotting confirmed that indeed his scotoma had contracted (Fig. 11). What had previously been a narrow crescent of residual amblyopic vision in the upper left quadrant (in an otherwise full macula-splitting homonymous hemianopa) had expanded into a region of apparently normal vision. There was also a slight contraction of the field defect along the lower vertical meridian. The resulting scotoma now occupied mainly the lower left quadrant, with some incursion into the upper quadrant in the central 30°–40°. The contracted scotoma was absolutely blind, according to D.B.'s report, when plotted with the largest brightest target in the Aimark perimeter (see above for stimulus parameters). The contracted scotoma has remained unchanged in size, shape, or density, within the limits of measurement, since 1976.

So much for an account of the clinical features of D.B.'s history. But it was very particular and unusual aspects of his visual capacity that brought him to our attention some six weeks after surgery. The ophthalmic surgeon at the National Hospital, Michael D. Sanders, noticed that D.B. appeared to be able to locate objects in his supposed blind field much more skilfully

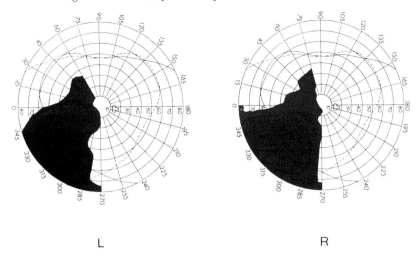

L   R

Fig. 11. D.B.'s contracted field defect 44 months postoperatively, measured on an Aimark perimeter, 1° 40′ target, high contrast. (Redrawn from Weiskrantz 1980, by permission)

than one might have expected. For example, even though D.B. could not see one's outstretched hand, he seemed to be able to reach for it accurately. We put movable markers on the wall to the left of his fixation, and again he seemed to be able to point to them, although he said he did not actually see them. Similarly, when a stick was held up in his blind field either in a horizontal or vertical position, and he was asked to guess which of these two orientations it assumed, he seemed to have no difficulty at all, although again he said he could not actually see the stick. After one such long series of 'guesses', when he made virtually no errors, he was told how well he had done. In the interview that followed, and which was recorded, D.B. expressed considerable surprise. 'Did you know how well you had done?', he was asked. 'No,' he replied, 'I didn't—because I couldn't see anything; I couldn't see a darn thing.' 'Can you say how you guessed—what it was that allowed you to say whether it was vertical or horizontal?' 'No, I could not because I did not see anything; I just don't know.' Finally, he was asked, 'So you really did not know you were getting them right?' 'No,' he replied, still with something of an air of incredulity.

This apparent dissociation between D.B.'s capacity and awareness of it we dubbed 'blindsight' (Sanders *et al.* 1974). In collaboration with Mr Sanders and Professor John Marshall (the neurologist in charge of D.B.'s case), we set out to study D.B.'s capacity more systematically and under better controlled conditions. Those findings were published and are available in detail (Weiskrantz *et al.* 1974), but for the sake of completeness and ease of reference are summarized here. (This first round of tests, in 1974, occurred well before the contraction of the scotoma.)

In all of the experimental procedures, which were carried out over two five-day periods, two to eight months post-operatively, D.B. was never given knowledge of results during the course of any experiment, although at the end of a series he was 'debriefed'. With the exception of the eye fixation experiment, which was carried out in a windowless room, all experiments were carried out in an office or in a corridor in which it was not possible to control the level of background lighting completely. During evening testing the conditions were just bright enough for us to record the results. Otherwise the lighting was made as dim as possible by not very effective venetian blinds. All testing in this early series was done binocularly.

Locating by eye fixation

The first procedure we carried out was an attempt to replicate the procedure and findings of Pöppel *et al.* (1973) in which they asked their subjects to move their eyes to the position in the blind field at which a light had flashed. D.B. was seated in the standard position in a Goldmann perimeter. He was told that a spot of light would be flashed in his blind field and, on a verbal signal, he was to shift his eyes from the standard fixation point to the position where he 'guessed' the spot had been projected. The largest stimulus size (2°) was used, at the brightest setting and the standard background luminance.

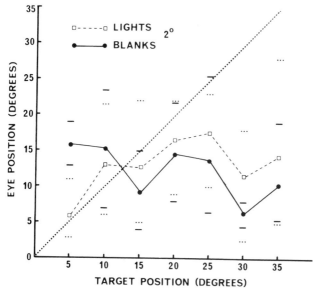

Fig. 12. Average eye positions for target positions of given eccentricity, presented in quasi-random order. For each target position, n = 5 for stimulus trials, and n = 3 for blanks. Bars above and below points indicate range of obtained eye positions. Dotted bars: stimulus trials. Solid bars: blank control trials. (Reprinted from Weiskrantz *et al.* 1974, by permission)

On each trial the stimulus was turned on for 3 seconds at a horizontal eccentricity of 5°, 10°, 15°, 20°, 25°, 30°, or 35° in random order. The spot was oscillated up and down by manual control over an arc of approximately 4° during each presentation. D.B. was asked to move his eyes only after the stimulus was extinguished, but not to move his head (which rested on a chin rest). In some series of trials half of the presentations were 'blanks', which were identical in all respects to the test trials except that the light was not turned on. D.B.'s eye position was measured conventionally with recording electrodes placed on the skin close to the eye. Typically, D.B. moved his eyes to the final 'steady state' position after two or three intermediary saccades. For present purposes only the 'steady state' position was used for analysis.

The results were similar to those of Pöppel *et al.* There was a weak but significant effect of target position on eye position (Fig. 12) out to an eccentricity of 25°. There was no significant control exercised by the 'blank' trials.

Locating by reaching with finger

The results of the eye fixation procedure were positive, but weak, and only held out to 25° eccentricity. It may be that it is unnatural to shift one's eyes more than this; typically over larger eccentricities one moves one's head and eyes. Meanwhile, we had been experimenting (see Chapter 1) with monkeys reaching with their hands to locate targets projected into their over wide eccentricities in defective fields, and the present experiment was roughly modelled on the same procedure. Also, we had carried out informal tests with D.B. using this method, and it seemed to be highly promising.

He was seated in the standard position for the Aimark perimeter. He was asked to maintain constant fixation within each trial on the fixation mark, and never to move his head. He was told that a spot of light would be flashed in the blind field for three seconds and afterwards, on a verbal signal, he was to reach with his forefinger to the guessed location of the spot without shifting his fixation. The spot was varied in size from 4° 15' to 23'. In some cases it was projected onto the perimeter arm from behind D.B. with a Keeler projector, and in others the Aimark projector target itself was used. All stimuli were projected along the horizontal meridian, the position randomly placed among six eccentricities from 15° to 90° (in 15° intervals). The series was presented in order of descending size, as indicated in Fig. 13a–d. Then, as a control for false cues, the largest size was given again (Fig. 13e), but with half the trials presented randomly as 'blanks'.

The results were striking for stimuli larger than 23' in diameter (Fig. 13), so much so that statistical analysis would be superfluous. In the final run, when 'blanks' were interjected randomly, his responses to the blanks were extremely variable and clearly different from the stimulus trials, in which

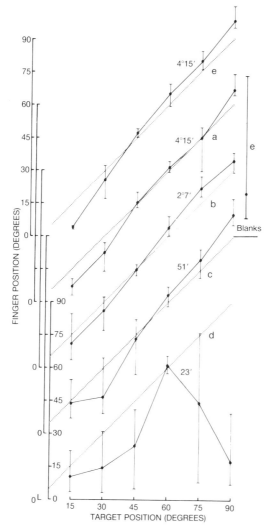

Fig. 13. Average finger reaching responses for targets of given eccentricity and diameter, presented in quasi-random order. Series was conducted in order **a** through **e**. Vertical bars indicate ranges of obtained values. For each point in conditions **a** to **d**, n = 6, in **e**, n = 3. In condition **e** blank trials (n = 18) were randomly interspersed between stimulus trials, and average response position and range for blanks are shown to right of experimental results. Dotted lines indicate slopes of functions for completely accurate responses. (Reprinted from Weiskrantz *et al.* 1974, by permission)

the position of the light continued to exercise a close control on where he reached. While the reaching was impressive, it was nevertheless not as accurate as in his good (right) half-field, where he was virtually perfect (Fig. 14), within the limits of measurement (to the nearest 0.5°).

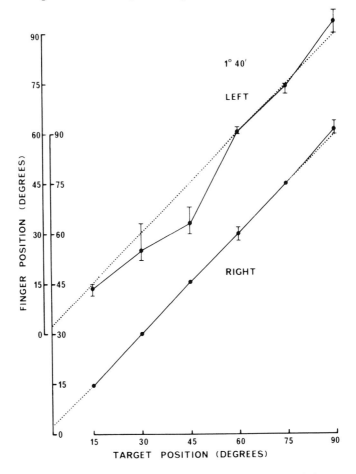

Fig. 14. Average finger reaching responses for 1° 40′ target of given eccentricity, n = 4 for each point. Vertical bars refer to ranges. The stimuli in right and left half-fields were randomly interspersed. (Reprinted from Weiskrantz *et al.* 1974, by permission)

Orientation of lines: vertical vs. horizontal, vertical vs. diagonal, and X vs. O

D.B. was seated in front of a projection screen. Projectors allowed us to flash a large variety of shapes onto the screen. Some of the runs consisted in requiring him to guess after each presentation whether a line was vertical or non-vertical. In another series, he was asked to guess whether the stimulus had been an 'X' or an 'O'. A shutter allowed the duration to be controlled. A large range of sizes and durations were used, as well as reversals of contrast (dark stimulus on white ground, or vice versa). The dimensions and durations

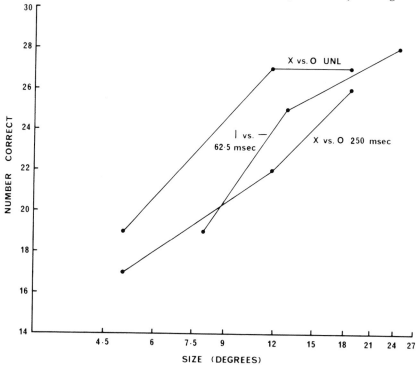

Fig. 15. The effect of size of stimulus on forced-choice performance. Size scale is logarithmic. Maximum score in all cases was 30; chance performance was 15. (From Weiskrantz *et al.* 1974, by permission)

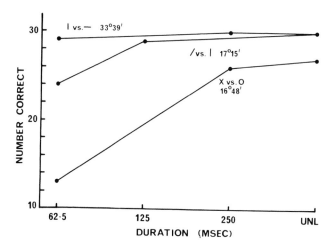

Fig. 16. The effect of duration on performance. Maximum score was 30; chance score was 15. UNL: unlimited duration, i.e., stimulus not extinguished until subject responded. (From Weiskrantz *et al.* 1974, by permission)

of the complete range of stimuli used are contained in the original report (Weiskrantz *et al.* 1974, Tables I and II) and are too numerous to reproduce here.

The results were clear. Both for orientation and 'shape', D.B. was able to guess correctly at well above chance levels, provided the stimuli exceeded a certain size and—if the discrimination was a difficult one—above a certain duration (see Figs. 15 and 16. In both figures, 30 correct is a perfect score). But with 'easy' discriminations, duration was virtually irrelevant; even at the short duration of 62.5 msec, he performed virtually perfectly. Nor did direction of contrast appear to matter. In the vertical vs. diagonal discrimination, the diagonal line was 27° 33′ off vertical, and this was clearly within his capability.

Acuity

It turned out that D.B. was able to guess whether or not a display contained a line-grating or not, and so it proved possible to measure his acuity, which was done for one eccentricity in his blind and his good fields. He was seated 53 cm in front of the apparatus, which contained diffraction gratings. When light was trans-illuminated through the apparatus, interference patterns were produced that approximated the configuration of a sine-wave grating. The width and separation of the bars in the grating (i.e., its spatial frequency) could be varied over a large range, without altering the total flux of the trans-illuminated field (details of the apparatus, originally used to measure monkeys' acuity, are in Weiskrantz and Cowey 1963). The grating field (6° 39′ in diameter) was placed so that its centre was 8° 48′ from the fixation point. D.B. was simply asked to respond 'lines' or 'no lines' (the 'no lines' condition being a grating of very high spatial frequency, equal in flux to all other settings, that appeared homogeneous in the good field) to a succession of stimuli presented singly.

Even though in his 'blind' field D.B. said he did not 'see' any lines, or indeed even the entire trans-illuminated field, which was quite bright—the light source was beamed through the diffraction plates from a Leitz projector (150 watts)—it was possible to obtain a measure of his minimal separable acuity (Fig. 17). In his good half-field (where, of course, he could always see the stimulus field) he was better than in his impaired field, but nevertheless his acuity in the latter was a creditable 1.9′ (or 15.8 cycles/degree).

Interestingly, the threshold in his amblyopic crescent was also measured and found to be just over 8′ (3.75 cycles/degree), which was considerably worse than the acuity in the blind field (which, of course, was measured at a point nearer the fixation point). Nevertheless, D.B. always reported 'seeing' the bars in the amblyopic remnant when they were above threshold (and always 'saw' the trans-illuminated field whether or not bars were visible in it) whereas he consistently reported seeing nothing, not even the bright field, in his blind region under any conditions of test.

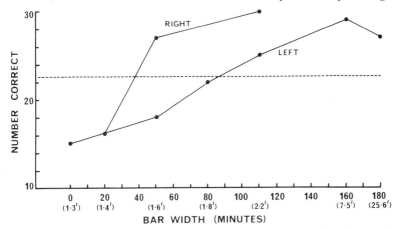

Fig. 17. Detection of a grating as a function of spatial separation of bars, from which 'minimal separable acuity' can be determined. Upper numbers on abscissa refer to calibration curve for apparatus in Weiskrantz and Cowey (1963, lower numbers to width of bar (or space)). Each point shows performance (maximum = 30) for given stimulus vs. narrowest bar width. Chance = 15. Dotted line shows 75% correct level. (From Weiskrantz *et al.* 1974, by permission)

Verbal commentaries

D.B. was questioned repeatedly about his vision in his left half-field. Most commonly he said that he saw nothing at all. If pressed, he might say in some tests, but by no means in all, that he perhaps had a 'feeling' that a stimulus was approaching or receding, or was 'smooth' (the **O**) or 'jagged' (the **X**). But always he stressed that he saw nothing in the sense of 'seeing', that typically he was guessing, and was at a loss for words to describe any conscious perception.

In his reporting, D.B. convinced us — and continued to do so throughout all subsequent studies — of his reliability and integrity as a reporter. If the projected stimulus happened to fall at the edge of the intact, crescent-shaped remnant of his left field he reported this promptly. If a bright stimulus was placed near the vertical meridian so that some light diffused into the good field, he also reported this promptly even if the effect was slight, and when asked to point to or describe the location of this visible light, always located it in the good field. At this early stage of testing, as mentioned above with his judgements of orientation of a stick, he often seemed openly surprised when he was told how well he had done. His intellectual curiosity about his own condition gradually grew, and he became, as it were, an interested observer of his own capabilities. He often reported his subjective responses to various visual situations in his everyday life that occurred between testing sessions, and continued to monitor the size of his field defect through informal, but quite accurate, procedures.

Tests since 1974

Since the original report in 1974 we have seen D.B. on a number of occasions, with a variety of procedures, but much remains unpublished. Some results were mentioned in a discussion (Weiskrantz 1978). Control procedures and some extensions of the earlier findings were summarized in a published review lecture (Weiskrantz 1980), and some findings on aspects of form perception and matching are in press (Weiskrantz and Warrington). It always seemed desirable to wait until yet another experiment could be done, and as D.B. lives some distance from London and Oxford, and also had to be compensated for loss of earnings, testing was intermittent. Meanwhile, however, the phenomenon of 'blindsight' has attracted a certain measure of publicity, interest, and speculation, and so it seems desirable at this time to gather together our observations made over several years, to place them on record, and to consider some of their possible implications.

Depending on varying practical and apparatus requirements, we tested him either in the National Hospital or in the Department of Experimental Psychology, Oxford, each on a number of occasions. We also tested him once at his home. Each testing session lasted 2 to 3 days.

The illumination and visual environmental conditions varied between occasions and locations, but since 1979 it has been possible to test him in a constant and controlled set-up, which is termed the 'standard situation' below; it is the same situation that has been used with a larger population of patients for comparative purposes.

For each type of psychophysical determination, D.B. was required to choose among a fixed set of alternatives or to reach along the arc of the Aimark perimeter set at a particular meridian. Alternatives were always presented according to random schedules prepared in advance (usually Gellerman schedules). If he was uncertain he was always required to guess. After each set of trials in any psychophysical run, he was asked to describe his subjective impressions of the stimuli and how well he thought he had performed, but knowledge of results was *never* given until the end of all testing for each 2–3 day session.

After January 1976, following the contraction of his field defect, psychophysical determinations were generally made along a meridian extending 30° or 45° below the horizontal in the lower left quadrant (using the lower right quadrant as control). Prior to that, testing had usually been along the horizontal meridian. Except where noted, all psychophysical testing was binocular. All light values were measured with an S.E.I. photometer, and we report the light values in the units in which that instrument is calibrated, log ft lamberts. (Conversion to candles/m^2 can be made by multiplying ft lamberts by 3.43.)

The methods and results for each category of psychophysical determination, together with the date it was carried out, are described in Part II.

Part II

3 Reaching for randomly located targets

Method

The general method (with one exception, see below) was always the same as that reported in our earlier study (Weiskrantz et al. 1974). D.B. was seated in the standard position for the Aimark perimeter, using the chin rest. He was asked to maintain constant fixation within each trial on the fixation mark, and never to move his head. He was told that, following a verbal 'ready' signal, a spot of light would be flashed in the blind field and afterwards, on a verbal signal, he was to reach with his forefinger to the guessed location of the spot without shifting his fixation. The duration of the target was two seconds, except (see below) when it was made much shorter for control purposes. The location of the teaching responses was measured by moving the target to the response position and reading directly from the scale. For any test run, the size and brightness of the stimulus was held constant, and its position randomly varied among a number of fixed positions (usually six positions, from 15° to 90° in 15° intervals).

In the standard situation (see Chapter 17), the background illumination was controlled and constant at approximately − 1.6 log ft lamberts, with the target intensity varying from − 0.58 to 1.2 log ft lamberts. The sizes could be varied from 10′ to 1° 40′ in diameter. But it was not always possible to maintain constant illumination in other situations, e.g., when testing was in D.B.'s home or in an office without black-out control.

This procedure has been run on at least 13 occasions since the original report in 1974. After January 1976, the meridian tested was always below the horizontal, running through the contracted field defect. The main purpose of the tests was to check, as a routine matter, whether D.B.'s ability to reach for targets in the blind field was retained over the years. In addition, an important aim was to control the duration of the target, the background illumination, to introduce random 'blank' trials, and to record eye position, so as to rule out possible artefacts due to stray light or other cues.

Results

D.B.'s capacity to reach to targets in his field defect has on the whole been well retained since 1974. In February 1975 a target whose position varied randomly along the horizontal meridian (1° 40′ diameter, 1.02 log ft lamberts, background − 1.18 log ft lamberts) was able to control his reaching, either with his left or right hand (cf. Table 1). Even a rather smaller and dimmer

Table 1   Reaching

Horizontal meridian

	Left hand						Right hand					
Target	15°	30°	45°	60°	75°	90°	15°	30°	45°	60°	75°	90°
Response	10°	25°	32°	56°	72°	90°	10°	26°	40°	57°	72°	85°
	8°	28°	40°	60°	75°	85°	15°	39°	40°	55°	68°	78°
Mean	9°	26.5°	36°	58°	73.5°	87.5°	12.5°	32.5°	40°	56°	70°	81.5°

(February 1975)

Table 2   Reaching

Horizontal meridian

	15°	30°	45°	60°	75°	90°
1° 40′ 0.5 log ft lamberts Mean R	15.6°	22.4°	19.2°	60.6°	68.4°	85.2°
50′ 0.0 log ft lamberts Mean R	22.2°	18.8°	28.6°	56.2°	68.2°	85°
33′ − 0.6 log ft lamberts Mean R	20.2°	18.2°	25.0°	56.6°	71.6°	88.4°
10′ − 0.6 log ft lamberts Mean R	21.6°	39.8°	40.2°	43.6°	54.2°	56.0°

(September 1975) n = 5 per position

Table 3   Reaching

Meridian 45° down

Targets	15°	30°	45°	60°	75°	90°
Mean R	12.5°	22.8°	35.8°	52.9°	66.5°	69.8°
Blanks	15°	30°	45°	60°	75°	90°
Mean R	33.2°	31.2°	32.0°	39.5°	38.2°	40.0°

(September 1979) n = 6 per position

target (10′ diameter, − 0.6 log ft lamberts) still maintained some control over his reaching (September 1975; Table 2). The background light level for the stimuli in Table 2 was − 1.8 log ft lamberts; the sizes and light values of the stimuli are shown in the table. An example of his responses four years later with a target (1° 40′ diameter, 1.18 log ft lamberts, − 1.5 log ft lamberts background) varied along the meridian 45° off horizontal can be seen in

Table 3. In this test, 50 per cent of the trials, randomly interspersed, were 'blanks', i.e., everything was identical to the target trials except that the light was not actually presented (the light was never actually switched off between trials but its path was blocked by slight and silent movement of a card just in front of the light source — well out of view of the subject).

As the principal meridian used for testing changed from horizontal to off-horizontal after January 1976, it is of interest to analyse the results for off-horizontal meridia tested prior to 1976. Unfortunately, this was done in only one session, and only briefly, in February 1975. When D.B. was switched abruptly from the horizontal to the meridian 45° off horizontal, his reaching fell to chance, but only 2 trials per locus were given. Later in the session, he switched from horizontal, to 15°, then to 30°, and finally to 45° off horizontal. The results are seen in Table 4 (light values the same as in Table 1). It is evident that he performed less well at non-horizontal meridia, but he was not random. Here again, only 2 trials per locus were given for each meridian. (The result for the 30° target position, horizontal meridian, is inexplicably anomalous. It was caused by one of the targets at this setting producing a single reaching response to 100°, almost 6 times more deviant from its target than any other response to any target.)

Table 4   Reaching

	15°	30°	45°	60°	75°	90°
Horizontal Mean R	15.0°	59.5°	36.0°	56.5°	71.0°	88.5°
15° meridian Mean R	34.0°	40.0°	43.0°	53.0°	72.0°	88.5°
30° meridian Mean R	42.0°	39.5°	39.5°	64.0°	71.0°	84.0°
45° meridian Mean R	29.5°	29.0°	55.0°	64.5°	66.0°	74.5°

(February 1975) n = 2 per position

He was tested for responses along a non-horizontal meridian briefly in the session immediately following the contraction of his field, but he was still complaining of interferences by spontaneous phosphenes, and so testing was not of much use. More thorough testing was carried out a month later, in February 1976, although unfortunately it had to be carried out under conditions under which it was impossible to maintain control of lighting conditions in the room (which was an office with varying amounts of light entering the windows). Early in the session we tried to compare his reaching along the horizontal meridian and a meridian 15° off-horizontal in the lower left quadrant. Because of the contraction of his field, this could not be done beyond 35° eccentricity. An attempt was made to block out light from the windows, resulting in a moderately dim illumination; the level was such that the stimuli were salient enough to produce an experience of 'something that came out towards me, darker than dark'. With the brightest Aimark target (50′ in diameter and 1.2 log ft lamberts) and testing in an ABBA order, he gave the results shown in Table 5 (6 trials per location). While there was a correlation between the mean reaching the target, the relationship was weak, and poorer than it had been in the past along the horizontal meridian. Later in the same session, when the room was a bit darker, he was tested again only along the meridian 15° off-horizontal, with the similar but slightly improved results shown in Table 6. On the following day, he was tested over a wider range of eccentricities along the 45° meridian off-horizontal in the lower left field, using the same size stimulus (50′) as in the previous tests, attenuated by 0.5 log units, and a moderately dim level of illumination. The results are shown in Table 7. His performance was inaccurate.

Table 5   Reaching

	Horizontal				15° Down			
	5°	15°	25°	35°	5°	15°	25°	35°
Mean R	10.1°	13.8°	16.0°	15.3°	8.6°	15.0°	18.8°	19.0°

(February 1976) n = 6 per position

Table 6   Reaching

Meridian 15° down				
Target	5°	15°	25°	35°
Mean R	10.1°	13.0°	18.0°	21.3°

(February 1976) n = 6 per position

Table 7   Reaching

Meridian 45° down						
Target	15°	30°	45°	60°	75°	90°
Mean R	39.1°	30.0°	41.8°	56.3°	47.3°	54.8°

(February 1976) n = 6 per position

Table 8   Reaching

Meridian 30° down						
Target	22°	37°	52°	67°	82°	97°
Mean R	29.7°	38.2°	51.3°	50.8°	55.0°	84.7°
Blanks Mean R	15.3°	12.8°	14.2°	12.5°	14.0°	12.2°

(April 1977) n = 6 per position

Thorough testing of a non-horizontal meridian (30°) in the lower left field after contraction of the scotoma was next carried out in April 1977. From the very outset his performance was good. The results for a run of 72 trials (half of them 'blanks') are shown in Table 8, also shown as 'Standard 2 sec' condition in Fig. 19. (The target was 1° 40′ diameter; ambient light level was not measured in this run, but was recorded as 'moderate' with a desk light on the floor shining upwards in the direction of the perimeter from behind D.B. From his verbal responses ['did not see anything. No movement, nothing at all. I seem to be aware of it in the periphery but centrally there was nothing at all'] we estimate a contrast with background of between 1 and 1.5 log units).

It is difficult to know just why D.B.'s responses were accurately controlled in this session (and thereafter), in contrast to the inaccurate pattern seen soon after the contraction of his field. The most likely reasons are the unstable character of his field soon after the contraction, with interfering effects of phosphenes, together with the practice that D.B. gave himself in his everyday life. He was an inveterate examiner of his own fields, and had a continuing interest in determining his accuracy in informal but sensible tests of his own devising.

Testing from 1979 onwards could be carried out under a standardized condition in a light-proof room. The background illumination on the perimeter arc was adjusted so that the largest-brightest target at an eccentricity

Table 9   Reaching

Meridian 45° down

Target	15°	30°	45°	60°	75°	90°
Mean R	23.3°	47.6°	51.0°	61.6°	49.3°	66.6°

Overhead light on:

Target	15°	30°	45°	60°	75°	90°
Mean R	32.0°	37.6°	54.0°	59.3°	70.0°	70.0°

(August 1983) n = 3 per position

Table 10   Reaching

Meridian 30° down

Target	15°	30°	45°	60°	75°	90°
Mean R	28.0°	41.2°	52.7°	57.7°	72.9°	84.2°

Meridian 45° down

Target	15°	30°	45°	60°	75°	90°
Mean R	11.5°	32.5°	47.0°	61.0°	58.5°	71.0°

(August 1983) n = 4 per position

of 15° produced no visible diffusion into the good field. Results for the first tests in this situation, along the 45° lower meridian, have already been presented above (Table 3).

In 1983 his reaching was studied under contrasting conditions of ambient illumination. In the standardized condition, he was tested with a 1° 40′ target (1.18 log ft lambers, background − 1.65 log ft lamberts) along the lower left 45° meridian, 3 trials per location. The same procedure was followed but with the overhead lights on, yielding a background level on the perimeter arc of 0.60 log ft lamberts (it also added 0.1 log unit to the light level of the target). The results are shown in Table 9. Testing was also carried out along both the 30° and 45° meridia on the next day under the standard conditions, 4 trials per location, with the results shown in Table 10. It will be seen that his reaching was obviously correlated with target position.

Control procedures

1. *Duration* of target: In a series of tests in September 1975, a camera shutter was fixed in front of the target light projector source of the Aimark perimeter; it was calibrated by means of a photo-cell and oscilloscope trace. As the minimum latency for initiation of a saccade is approximately 150 msec, even had D.B. moved his eyes after the onset of the target to bring it on to a good portion of his field, the target would no longer have been present with the two durations tested, 125 msec and 67 msec. Figure 18 shows the results of testing (5 trials per location) along the horizontal meridian with

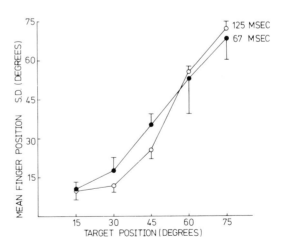

Fig. 18. Mean (S.D. in brackets) locations of reaching responses by D.B. in Aimark perimeter for randomly presented 1° 40′ target of brief duration presented along horizontal meridian. Stimulus brightness 0.5 log ft lamberts against perimeter background of − 1.6 log ft lamberts, with screen behind of − 1.0 log ft lamberts. Weiskrantz and Warrington, unpublished data recorded on 19/9/75. (From Weiskrantz 1980, by permission)

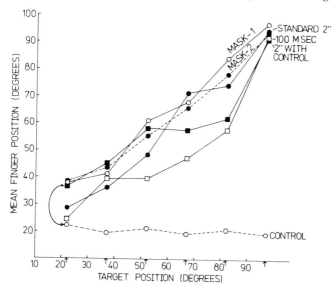

Fig. 19. Mean reaching responses by D.B. in Aimark perimeter. Standard condition: 1° 40′ target presented for 2 sec, fixation maintained throughout. Control: reaching responses to 'blank' stimuli in which settings, etc., were same as in experimental trials, but no targets were presented. Control trials were randomly interspersed and comprised 50% of trials. Mask-1: screen behind perimeter arc set at 2.55 log ft lamberts; perimeter arc at 0.6 log ft lamberts, and target spot at 1.3 log ft lamberts. Mask-2: screen behind perimeter arc at 2.55 log ft lamberts, perimeter arc in intact visual field at 2.8 log ft lamberts, arc in 'blind' field at 1.0 log ft lamberts, and target at 1.3 log ft lamberts. Stimuli presented along meridian 30° below horizontal. Weiskrantz and Warrington, unpublished data, recorded on 22/4/77. (From Weiskrantz 1980, by permission)

a 2° target (target 0.5 log ft lamberts; background − 1.6 log ft lamberts). After the contraction of the scotoma, a similar test (10 trials per location) was carried out for targets along a meridian 30° off-horizontal, with a duration of 100 msec, and with stimulus/ambient light levels the same as with Table 5. The results are shown in Fig. 19. It is clear that adventitious eye movements cannot account for the reaching performance.

2. Eye movement recordings: Throughout the whole of the runs plotted in Fig. 18 eye position was monitored continuously by means of an infra-red detecting device mounted on spectacle frames designed by Heywood and Churcher (unpublished; we are indebted to the late Dr S. Heywood and Mr J. Cole for their assistance with this phase of the experiment). Records of the first and last eight trials of a 30-trial session with a target duration of 125 msec are shown in Fig. 20, together with the position of each target and response during those trials. It is clear that D.B.'s visual fixation is very stable and well controlled, even during the reaching response itself, and that

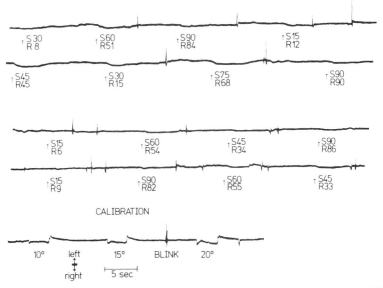

Fig. 20. Continuous eye movement recordings during first and last eight trials of a 30-trial session in which D.B. reached to location along horizontal meridian at which target had appeared in Aimark perimeter in his 'blind' field. S: target location. R: response location, in degrees from fixation. Arrow: time of target presentation. Target size and light values as in Fig. 18, duration 125 msec. Weiskrantz and Warrington, unpublished data, recorded on 19/9/75. (From Weiskrantz 1980, by permission)

fixation reflexes cannot account directly for his accuracy in locating the stimuli.

3. Flooding of surround field: Because the field defect, especially after it has contracted, was surrounded by a large intact field of vision, it is important to rule out artefacts due to diffusion of light within the eye onto the good field and also artefacts due to reflections among surfaces in the room. The former can be controlled entirely, and the latter to a large extent, by flooding the intact field with light levels sufficiently intense so that even were there to be stray light from the target into the intact field it would not be detectable. The arrangement used (in April 1977) was the following: A large white screen (approximately 3 feet wide by 2.5 feet high) was placed approximately 2 feet behind the perimeter. Black cardboard was cut to the size and shape of the field defect, and was placed immediately behind the perimeter arm so as to mask the scotoma from the white screen behind it. Two powerful photo-flood lamps were placed to shine on to the white screen and partially on to the perimeter screen (Mask-1). In a second condition (Mask-2), a piece of white cardboard was fixed on to the whole of the portion of the perimeter screen that fell within the intact field, so as to raise its brightness.

Under these conditions, one can say that diffusion is reduced to negligible levels. Even ignoring the illuminated background screen, a spot of 0.3 log units more intense than the background of the perimeter arc (as in the Mask-2 condition) can be increased in diameter to about 2.8° and still be completely invisible when projected on to the optic disc, i.e., detectable intra-ocular diffusion can be no more than the order of 1°, as a conservative estimate. Considered in relation to the background screen, diffusion is negligible. In a simulation experiment, we projected a spot of the same size and initial brightness as in the Mask-2 condition directly on to a screen raised to a light level of 2.5 log ft lamberts, as in the Mask-2 condition. Under those conditions the spot was not measurably brighter than the background with the S.E.I. photometer, although it could just be detected when viewed foveally. It could not be seen at all, even when flickering, at an eccentricity of 15° (3 observers). And so, even if it had been reflected without any degradation whatever into the good field, it could not possibly suffice to direct reaching with the accuracy shown by D.B. His results are shown in Fig. 19.

4. *'Monkey perimeter' and verbal responding:* To ensure that D.B.'s performance was not restricted to just one type of apparatus, in April 1977 we used a hemi-spherical dome originally designed to plot visual fields of animals (Cowey and Weiskrantz 1963). Independent target lights (1° diameter) are mounted on a 5° by 5° grid. A schematic drawing of the stimulus array is shown in Fig. 21. In addition, 4 large 'background' floodlights were mounted within the perimeter and directed towards the screen to raise the level of illumination (in the tests with D.B., with one exception, we used only two such lamps, I and II in Fig. 21), and in a further condition two photo-flood lamps were mounted directly behind the D.B. to raise the level of the right half and upper left half of the dome. A reaching response was possible in the apparatus, but it was more convenient—and of interest in its own right—to instruct D.B. to use a verbal response. He was asked to say 'top' if he guessed the briefly lit target was near the fixation point, and 'bottom' if it was more peripheral. In another condition, he discriminated among three possible targets, by responding 'near', 'middle', or 'far' (stimuli marked 'A', 'F', and 'B', respectively, in Fig. 21), with an ambient background of 1.1 log ft lamberts. The situation was more difficult, partly, no doubt, because of using a forced choice among three alternatives, with some verbal confusion intruding as well. He scored 60 per cent overall in 180 trials (chance = 33 per cent). In a control condition for inadvertent non-visual cues, when the background level within the lower left quadrant was raised by turning all four background floodlights, thereby substantially reducing the contrast virtually to zero, his performance fell to chance (13/30). Otherwise, under the ambient background condition of 1.1 log ft lamberts, he scored on average better than 90 per cent when using a forced choice between 2 alternatives ('top' vs. 'bottom'), the performance depending on the separation between

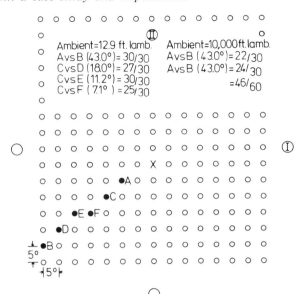

Fig. 21. Scheme of stimulus bulbs set within hemisphere of 'monkey perimeter'. D.B. was asked to report 'top' if target fell nearer to fixation point, and 'bottom' if farther from fixation point. Inset shows various discriminations and distances between pairs of targets in degrees, with numbers correct out of 30 with forced-choice procedure. I and II indicate photo-flood lamps set within dome; there were also two powerful photo-flood lamps behind subject to control ambient levels. Ambient levels refer to portion of dome in intact visual fields. Target: 68′ diameter, 2 sec duration, 4 log ft lamberts. Weiskrantz and Warrington, unpublished data, recorded on 23/4/77. (From Weiskrantz 1980, by permission)

stimuli, but even for two targets separated by just 7° of visual angle he scored 83 per cent.

The level of illumination of the intact field could be raised to very high levels without abolishing D.B.'s ability to discriminate position. In the most extreme condition, with two photo-floods and two apparatus background floodlights on, the level in the right half of the dome reached the maximum measurable level with the photometer (4 log ft lamberts), and his performance still remained above chance. (Under these extreme conditions, there was also some increase in ambient level of the lower left quadrant, thereby reducing the contrast.) A summary of the conditions and results is given in Fig. 21.

Verbal commentaries

As mentioned above, after most runs (typically of 30 or 60 forced-choice trials) D.B. was asked to report any subjective experience he had felt, and also to say how well he thought he had performed, and with what confidence. He became quite accustomed to giving us reports of his introspections and of his daily experiences in relation to his blind field—and also of any detectable stray light or any other mishaps in the set-ups. In the Aimark reaching experiments, our impression is that over the years he gradually became more likely to report having a certain type of experience, difficult to describe, for stimuli of high contrast, long duration, and rapid onset/offset, or movement. The experience was also more likely to be felt with stimuli in certain parts of the scotoma. Thus, after reaching to a high contrast and large set of stimuli along the 30° off-horizontal meridian the exchange went as follows: 'Q: How well did you do? A: I think with the ones out here [pointed to the peripheral part of the perimeter] I did pretty well. Q: But did you see the light? A: No, I didn't see anything. Q: Did you see any movement? A: No. Q: Did you see *anything*? A: No, nothing at all. I seem to know or be aware of it in the periphery but centrally I would say there was nothing at all.' He always firmly denied having any visual experience as such, but with very salient stimuli he was apt to say 'They all appeared to stand out in front of the screen. I felt I could push them back' (September 1979). Nor, it should be stressed, was the periphery of the field always favoured along all meridia. On the other hand, the occurrence of such an experience was not necessarily associated with accurate reaching. On the occasion in February 1976, when he was tested on the lower 45° off-horizontal meridian soon after his scotoma had contracted (Table 7), he also commented that he had 'the same feeling of a billiard cue as yesterday (i.e., the results shown in first table for that day) but not so strong'. Nevertheless his reaching performance was not accurate.

As the salience was decreased, so the likelihood and strength of such an experience was reduced. Thus, in April 1977, when the duration was reduced to 100 msec, with no change in contrast or size, he said 'I am not aware of anything at all. Q: How did you do? A: It was pure guess work'. (This for the results shown in Fig. 19). As the size and contrast were reduced but duration held constant at two seconds in the same session, he said they 'no longer came out as far', and with weakest stimuli in that set, 'a couple of times I felt they were there, but not so powerful a feeling to make me *know* they were there'.

His comment during the 1979 testing (Table 3) was 'all the stimuli stood out from the perimeter about 3 inches'.

The 1983 tests (Tables 9 and 10) when he seemed to have quite 'lively' regions of his field, yielded the comment 'I have a feeling of a quick movement out to about 45°' [pointing to the perimeter arc]. When the overhead lights were turned on, so that there was only a 0.6–0.7 log unit difference between the target and ground, he nevertheless said he had the same kind of experience as in the dimmer condition 'but not so prominent. It was live out to about 30°' [again pointing to perimeter arc]. When tested again in the dimmer ambient condition along the 30° and 45° meridia (Tables 8 and 9), he said, 'There was a definite movement. Something seems to pop out a couple of inches'. Pressed further to describe it, he said, 'I did not see any light. If anything it was a sort of dark. A moving wave'. Similarly, in the 'monkey perimeter, when the contrast was increased by turning off the internal perimeter flood-lamps, he said 'I felt as if something was coming up to me. But I didn't *see* anything'. But when the contrast was reduced (results in Fig. 19) and with maximal flooding of the intact field, when his performance was well above chance, he said in response to what he had felt, 'Nothing at all. Just guessing. No feelings of anything. No idea at all'.

Further treatment of these commentaries will be taken up in Part III. Here it is worth stressing that D.B. was adamant that his 'feelings' could not be simulated by any experience of stimuli presented to the good visual field, even in the very far periphery, nor were they ever 'seeing'. Another point is that the success of his performance did not depend on his having any experience whatever — he still did well when he judged that he was 'guessing', even when pressed and despite his fluency and cooperation in giving introspective reports. There were other occasions when he had definite 'feelings' of 'something coming out', and yet performed poorly.

4   'Presence' vs. 'absence'

The question of D.B.'s capacity for detecting the presence of a visual stimulus has been examined by us on at least ten occasions. The main questions have concerned his sensitivity as a function of size, intensity, duration of the visual stimulus, and its location in the visual field. As in the study of reaching, before 1976 the meridian tested was always the horizontal one, and after the contraction of his field defect a meridian off-horizontal in the lower left quadrant was used.

Of all the capacities we have tested, this one presents the greatest danger of possible artefacts caused by incidental cues, and, in fact, we have never published results on detection sensitivity before now because of wishing to assure ourselves on this issue. Unlike the other tests, where the subject is asked to choose between two alternative values of a stimulus or one of a number of alternative locations, here he is only asked to detect its presence. The alternative stimulus is non-detection, and 'blank' control trials are simply further examples of this alternative, and hence are meaningless unless one gives an entire block of trials as blanks, which raises other difficulties if done more than occasionally. We have, in fact, done this on various occasions, and have discovered how careful one must be, for example, about the silence of the switching for the positive vs. negative stimuli or any other event that correlates with the presentation of the stimulus. We discovered, for example, that the 'silent' control switch on the Aimark is silent to the operator but not invariably to the subject, with his head in contact with the chin rest, and so we abandoned all data in which that switching method was used in which satisfactory control runs were not carried out. Here we present only those findings in which we are satisfied that there was a genuine discrimination of a signal vs. blanks. We have excluded any runs where we were uncertain on this point, (but no such data would alter our conclusions even had they been included). Another point is that, as with any 'go–no-go' procedure, performance levels are probably more susceptible to variation with fatigue and activation; with changing false-positive rates for the negative stimuli, the chance level of performance for positive stimuli will also vary. Finally, with tests of detection, when the subject need respond only to any feature of the stimulus, the problem of stray light affecting an intact part of the field is more serious than, say, orientation or acuity, where the critical feature to be discriminated is degraded with straying. D.B., in fact, was absolutely punctilious in reporting any stray light into an intact area of his field, but nevertheless the safe limits are more severe than with 'presence' vs. 'absence' than with other discriminations.

We also came to realize that the procedure of randomly changing the location of the stimulus from trial to trial, which is necessarily always done in experiments with reaching, was not the best way to test detection. More reliable findings are obtained, as will be seen, if the location is kept constant for a block of trials and the subject asked to make forced-choice, 'present/absent' responses within that block, before moving to a new location and a further block, and the subject is told at which location the critical events will take place. It seems reasonable to explain this advantage in terms of focusing of attention to a position in the 'blind' field.

Our results were obtained principally in two situations: stimuli presented in the Aimark perimeter, or presented on a screen by a projecting tachistoscope.

Aimark perimeter

In various pilot presence vs. absence studies carried out in 1975, prior to the contraction of his field defect, we reached the tentative conclusion that along the horizontal meridian or the meridian 15° below horizontal, D.B. was rather more sensitive to stimuli eccentrically located than more centrally located, just opposite to the gradient seen in his normal intact half-field. This was of interest because of the speculation that the 'second visual system' might be biased towards peripheral vision. We also concluded, with greater certainty, that his left eye was more sensitive than his right, a point in which we were interested because, as a result of his right cervical sympathectomy in 1970 (Weiskrantz *et al.* 1974), his right pupil was more constricted than his left. Thus, when the two eyes were tested at a point 60° eccentric along the left horizontal meridian (target 1° 40', light level of 0.78 log ft lamberts, perimeter background of − 1.7 log ft lamberts, background screen behind perimeter of − 1.1 log ft lamberts), he was perfect with his left (30/30), but not quite as good with his right eye (26/30, no false positives). When the intensity of the target was reduced by almost 1.0 log unit (to − 0.18 log ft lamberts, with the background still at − 1.7 log ft lamberts), and its diameter reduced to 50', he still made only one error out of 30 with his left eye (not a false positive), but dropped to 20/30 with his right eye (4 false positives).

In February 1976, soon after the contraction of the field, he was tested on various meridia running through the lower left quadrant, but concentrating on the 45° meridian. The results of the tests with that meridian are shown in Table 11, in the order in which they were carried out. Initial intensity was 0.5 log ft lamberts against a background estimated to be − 1.0 log ft lamberts. Size was held constant within blocks of 20 trials, within which eccentricity was varied randomly from 15° to 75° in 15° intervals. Sizes across blocks varied from 1° 40' to 33'. D.B. performed at about threshold levels (65 per cent and 75 per cent respectively) for the largest and the intermediate target sizes. When the size was further reduced, his performance fell to chance (10/20), and did not recover until a larger and more intense (1.15 log ft lamberts) target was used.

Table 11   Presence/absence

Meridian 45° down

	Intensity (log ft lamberts)	15°	30°	45°	60°	75°	False positives
1° 40'	0.5	2/2	2/2	2/2	1/2	1/2	3/10
50'	0.5	2/2	2/2	2/2	0/2	0/2	3/10
33'	0.5	1/2	0/2	1/2	0/2	1/2	3/10
1° 40'	0.5	2/2	2/2	2/2	1/2	2/2	8/10
1° 40'	1.15	2/2	2/2	2/2	2/2	2/2	6/10
	Total	9/10	8/10	9/10	4/10	6/10	23/50

(February, 1976)

But, contrary to our pilot studies along the horizontal or near-horizontal meridia, detection along the 45° meridian showed a bias towards the more central loci, as one would expect for the intact half-field. The results were even more pronounced if only the performance runs are considered in which D.B. performed above chance (75 per cent, 70 per cent, and 65 per cent): in these cases, *all* the detection failures (false negatives) were at the 60° and 75° eccentricities.

But given the variability of the results when the location of the target was randomly varied from trial to trial, in April 1977 we decided to change to a modified 'Latin square' type of design in which D.B. was given blocks of 20 trials with eccentricity and target parameters held constant within each block. The rationale was that he would not be required continuously to change his focus of attention, as in the previous tests. Before each block he was shown where the target would appear in the field defect. This method was first used for the lower left 30° meridian. Target parameters were varied in the order shown in Table 12. The target duration was again two seconds. The setting of the Aimark arc was -0.4 log ft lamberts. Over all blocks the size varied from 1° 40′ to 33′ and the light value of the target from 1.15 log ft lamberts to 0.2 log ft lamberts. The table shows the percentage correct for all stimulus trials combined, both positive and blanks, as well as the false positive rate for negative stimuli separately (in brackets). Using this procedure, it was confirmed that, indeed, under these conditions D.B. was superior in peripheral vision than in central vision along this meridian, 30° off-horizontal, in contrast to the results for the 45° meridian, but in agreement with our earlier pilot results. (It should be noted that, under the conditions of this test, all stimuli fell within the field defect as defined by whether he reported seeing them. The limits of the field defect shown in Figs. 10 and 11 were obtained deliberately using a substantially higher contrast level to produce the most conservative limits, cf. Chapter 2.)

Table 12   Presence/absence

Meridian 30° down

	Intensity (log ft lamberts)	37°		52°		67°		82°	
1° 40′	1.15	57.5%	(35%)	40%	(50%)	92.5%	(5%)	87.5%	(0%)
33′	0.2	55	(40)	55	(35)	47.5	(45)	60	(40)
50′	0.2	42	(50)	45	(60)	90	(0)	100	(0)
50′	−0.2	55	(50)	40	(70)	40	(60)	40	(70)

(April 1977)

In order to show that this is not an idiosyncrasy of either the situation or of D.B.'s normal vision, a further Latin square procedure was run for the intact field, but because he was at ceiling with the weakest target that had been used in the left field, the target size was reduced to 10′ diameter and the intensity to -0.55 log ft lamberts; background luminance on the perimeter arc was moderately lower at -0.9 log ft lamberts. The result was that D.B. performed perfectly at 37° and 52° eccentricity, and at chance (50 per cent) at 67° and 82° (n = 20 per locus), conforming to a normal gradient of sensitivity with field position under these conditions.

Finally, in September 1979 it was possible to make a direct comparison between the 45° and 30° off-horizontal meridia. Using a Latin square design, and with blocks of 10 trials presented at eccentricities from 30° to 75°, in 15° intervals, a series was run for the 45° meridian with decreasing size and intensity of the target, with a background level on the perimeter arc of − 1.6 log ft lamberts. The duration of the target was two seconds. Then a Latin square procedure was run with one of the supra-threshold target settings for the 30° meridian. The stimulus values and results were shown in Table 13. It will be seen that the two gradients were opposite in slope. For the 30° meridian, as was also true of the horizontal meridian, the trend is for increasing sensitivity with increasing eccentricity. For the 45° meridian, running more or less through the centre of the field defect, the more peripheral loci were less sensitive than the more central ones, conforming also to the gradient seen in the normal half-field.

Table 13   Presence/absence

Meridian 45° down

	Intensity (log ft lamberts)	30°	45°	60°	75°
1° 45′	1.18	100%	100%	100%	100%
(n = 10 per location)					
50′	1.18	97.5	87.5	82.5	77.5
(n = 40 per location)					
50′	0.78	85	30	40	40
(n = 40 per location)					

Meridian 30° down

	Intensity (log ft lamberts)	30°	45°	60°	75°
50′	1.18	70	85	82.5	90

(September 1979)

Thus, it seems that along the 45° meridian, running through the heart of the scotoma, a normal gradient of sensitivity is found, with a reversed gradient at more peripheral meridia. This finding, which probably reflects varying densities of deficit, will be discussed further in Part III.

Verbal commentaries

In the Aimark perimeter, for stimuli of high contrast he typically said that although he did not 'see' anything 'I said "yes", when I thought there was something there. It was like something coming out from the surface'.

Similarly, he said that 'sometimes it is like a billiard cue coming out or going back, and when that happens I say "yes" '. It was often possible to relate his comments to specific field positions when using the Latin square design, and in general his level of performance was correlated with the likelihood of his making comment of this sort. Under some conditions he seemed to be more impressed by something 'going back' at the end of the trial, than by its 'going forward' at the beginning. At the two more peripheral loci shown in Table 13, he tended to say they were going back, and for the inner two loci, going forward. The same was true for both the lower left 45° and 30° degree meridia, even though the two performance functions were opposite in slope.

There were some performances, however, in which he reported no such experiences and yet performed well. There were several instances in earlier pilot studies (not reported here) in which he said he was 'purely guessing'. Thus, in examining him in 1976 with targets at 25° and 35° on the horizontal and 15° meridia, his performance was 86 per cent over 56 trials throughout which said it was 'pure guess-work'. Similarly, in the comparison of the 30° and 45° meridia in September 1979, using a Latin square design, in many of the blocks he was it was 'all guessing', even when his performance was above chance. For example, in the last block he scored 80 per cent out of 30 trials (for the 45° eccentricity on the 30° meridian) in which he denied having any experience.

Projecting tachistoscope

The stimulus was always a circular disc, 10° in diameter, projected onto a darker ground. The set-up used was always that of the 'standard situation' (see Chapter 17), in which all quadrants being tested were flooded by two projectors each. The duration of the stimulus was always 150 msec.; only the 45° meridian in the lower quadrant has been tested.

Where threshold runs were made, it was always by the modified stair-case method, with an intensity step interval of 0.2 log units, starting with a level four or more steps above presumed or measured threshold. In September 1979, after completing the standard measurements, which are always at 25° eccentricity on the 45° off-horizontal meridian, we proceeded to examine his performance at various eccentricities along that meridian.

We first examined his capacity at an eccentricity of 45°, using a target of 1.84 log ft lamberts, with a background light level of in the test quadrant of −1.05 log ft lamberts. The other three quadrants had levels of 0.40 log ft lamberts. He performed at 96.7 per cent correct out of 30 trials. We then illuminated not only the other three quadrants with projectors (yielding a level on them of 0.40 log ft lamberts), but also the area immediately below and adjacent to the target position by two projectors (light values not measured, but estimated to be 0.40 log ft lamberts, as the projectors were the same as illuminated the other quadrants), effectively reducing contrast substantially, and he performed at 27/30. Next, we directed one projector just below and another immediately to the left of the disc position, and he again performed at 27/30. Keeping the projectors in that position, we then reduced the intensity of the disc to 1.0 log ft lamberts, and he fell to chance (16/30). Upon raising it to the 1.84 level again, he performed at 10/10. Next, in order to reduce a possible slight effect of reflection from his nose, we applied dark face powder and cream, and he performed at 29/30 (i.e., as will be explained in Chapter 17) this effective reduction of 0.3 log units did not affect his performance). Finally, still with face powder on his nose we reduced the light value of the disc to 1.34 log ft lamberts, and he performed at 80 per cent (24/30). Reduced still further by another 0.2 log units, he fell to 18/30, and when the 0.2 log units were then restored, he once again performed at 24/30. And so his threshold lay between 1.34 and 1.14 log ft lamberts, against its own background of approximately 2.3 log units dimmer than the target and an immediately neighbouring background approximately 0.8 log units dimmer than the target.

Later we measured his threshold using the modified staircase method at eccentricities between 45°, 35°, 25°, 20°, and 15°, in that order. Finally we went through the same procedure in the same order for the good field, for the 45° off-horizontal meridian in the lower right quadrant. The results can be seen in Fig. 22, curve D. (In the figure, 0 attenuation is measured from a value of 1.84 log ft lamberts). It will be seen that once again his sensitivity along this 45° meridian, unlike that found for the horizontal or 30°

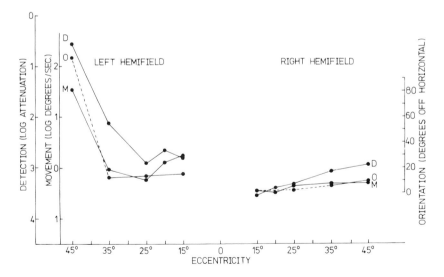

Fig. 22.   Thresholds for detection (D), orientation (O), and movement (M), as a function of eccentricity for left and right hemifields. (See text for conditions)

off-horizontal meridia (see Chapter 4), is poorer in peripheral than in central vision, as is also true of the good field. It can be seen that his threshold rises rather sharply between 35° and 45° eccentricity.

In April 1982, we were able to measure his threshold again, using the same staircase procedure in the 'standard situation' set-up, for the same 10° disc at an eccentricity of 45° on the 45° off-horizontal meridian. His threshold was found to be 1.37 log ft lamberts, virtually the same as his threshold more than 20 months earlier (1.28 log ft lamberts).

Threshold measurements were also made along the 60° off-horizontal meridian, but only for eccentricities of 25° and 35°. The staircase method was used, under the same conditions as above. At 25° his threshold was 2.85 log units of attenuation below the reference point, and at 35° it was 1.22 log units of attenuation, showing the same direction of gradient as the 45° meridian (see Fig. 22) and roughly of the same order of magnitude.

Detection was also measured routinely in the standard situation but only at one fixed eccentricity. The results will appear below (Chapter 17). We also measured his sensitivity with much smaller stimuli when plotting the optic disc and neighbouring points in the scotoma, and these results appear in Chapter 10.

Verbal commentaries

Throughout the whole set of procedures in which his capacity was tested with the projecting tachistoscope at 45° eccentricity, he said he 'was guessing all the way. I am not sure of anything'. For example, immediately after performing at 29 out of 30 he said, 'Just guessing. I don't think I did very well'. This same type of comment was also made when the 45° point was repeated with the staircase method: he said he was 'guessing all the way through', even though he started out performing perfectly (18/18) at the start of the descent of the staircase. He made exactly the same type of comment at 35° eccentricity ('No idea. I was just guessing; did not do very well'.) even though here the sensitivity was better by some 1.5 log units than it was at 45° (i.e. 0.8 log ft lamberts above background level in the lower left test quadrant, and actually *dimmer* than the ambient level of the other 3 quadrants by more than 0.5 log units). From an eccentricity of 25° inwards, however, he 'did not see', but had the impression of some 'little curved waves coming out from the wall about half an inch.' He also said of these eccentricities that he 'started out doing well, but then ended up guessing', which would fit the sequence in the staircase which started with stimulus values more than 1 log unit above threshold.

Comment

Through the heart of the field defect, his sensitivity is depressed, but it follows the same direction of gradient as in the normal, good field. While detection measurements are the most susceptible to artefacts either through stray light or adventitious cues, we see no reason to doubt the threshold measurements obtained here. As regards stray light, it is difficult to extrapolate to our situations from the values recommended by Wilson (1968) to protect against detection due to scattered light, because of the difference in conditions. Calculations for some of our experiments using Wilson's formula fall very far below his unsafe lower limit (e.g., Table 13, where the ratio of the target to background luminance × (target diameter)^2 is only 4.2, with an 85 per cent level of performance, and Table 12, where the calculation is only 1.11 for performances of 90 per cent and 100 per cent), but unfortunately he does not provide estimates for our lower levels of ambient illumination. These low contrast levels, however, together with the safe limit procedure outlined in the standard situation, plus the fact that D.B. carried out discriminations (e.g., location, orientation) under much higher levels ambient illumination and with low contrast, which hence must have been capable of detection *per se*, make it reasonable cautiously to accept the results here as fair estimates of his sensitivity within the scotoma. And, as with other discriminations, his capacity does not depend upon an acknowledged experience.

5   Visual acuity

In our original report (Weiskrantz *et al.*, 1974), we used an Ives apparatus that generates a sine-wave grating when light is passed through a pair of diffraction gratings (Moiré fringes; the apparatus is the same as that described more fully in Weiskrantz and Cowey 1963). Only one position in the scotoma was tested originally. The grating was visible in a circular aperture, 6° 39′ diameter, which was placed so that its centre was either 8° 48′ to the left or right of the fixation point (53 cm from the subject), depending on which visual half-field was being tested. Stimuli were presented singly, and D.B. was asked to report 'lines' or 'no lines', and the spatial frequency varied randomly from trial to trial so that a threshold determination could be made. Even though D.B. reported not only seeing no lines at all, but not even the brightly lit aperture, his performance varied systematically with the spatial frequency, and an acuity threshold could be determined. The results are summarized in Fig. 17 in Part I, where it can be seen that his minimal separable acuity in the impaired field at this position was a creditable 15.8 cycles/degree, as compared with 20 cycles/degree in the mirror symmetric region of the intact right half-field.

Here an extension is reported in which acuity was estimated as a function of retinal eccentricity, especially as the original determinations were made with the nearest edge of the grating only 5° 28′ from the fixation point. Also, because the Ives interference apparatus itself appears as a luminous source (light from a lamp immediately behind the two diffraction plates is passed through the plates), we thought it important also to test acuity using non-luminous, non-projected stimuli. For this purpose, photographic prints were also prepared of sine wave gratings generated on an oscilloscope and the prints, mounted on cardboard, were presented under conditions of normal overhead fluorescent room illumination. All measurements were made along the horizontal meridian, before the scotoma had contracted.

With both sets of stimuli, the procedure was the same. D.B. was presented randomly either with a grating of a given spatial frequency (contrast was constant throughout) or a plain stimulus matched in flux. (Actually, the 'plain' stimulus was always one of very high spatial frequency, well beyond the resolving power of any subject, to ensure that the flux was matched). The stimulus duration was not rigidly controlled, but was usually about three seconds. He was provided with a fixation point at varying angular separations from the stimulus. D.B. was asked to respond 'lines' or 'no lines' on each trial, and guessing was encouraged. Spatial frequency was varied after groups of 30 trials and acuity was calculated to be the interpolated value of cut-off spatial frequency that would yield a performance level of 75 per cent (chance being 50 per cent).

Ives apparatus, central 30 degrees

The apparatus was at a fixed distance from the frontal plane of 40.6 cm. Testing was carried out in D.B.'s home (October 1974), and it was not possible to control ambient illumination throughout the course of each day, but the brightness of the grating produced by the Ives apparatus is relatively independent of ambient illumination. Its value was 2.0 log ft lamberts for a setting of a spatial frequency so high that it was invisible to the normal field, and this value did not vary by a measurable amount over the range of ambient conditions actually used. The total flux of the trans-illuminated field and the contrast of the grating are independent of spatial frequency. The contrast of the grating was 78 per cent [100 × (peak − trough)/(peak + trough)]. Under dimmer ambient conditions, however, the contrast between the overall grating itself and the background was greater, and it appeared, to a normal observer, as a more distinctive stimulus. It is also worth noting that the total flux of the grating was less in the present series than in our 1974 study, where we had used a Leitz Type 31 044 000, 150 watt slide projector with an Elmaron lens as a light source, instead of an ordinary 100 watt household bulb. Using a Latin square design, D.B. was presented with groups of 30 trials in which the nearest edge of the grating was 6.25°, 16.5°, or 25.8°

eccentric from fixation, and the setting of the apparatus held constant at one of three different settings of number of cycle across the diameter of the grating aperture (9, 45, or 75 cycles) for each block of 90 trials. The grating aperture was 6.35 cm. Because the angular size of the grating aperture changed slightly with eccentricity in this condition, with all positions in the frontal

Table 14   Acuity—left field

	Eccentricity		
	6.25°	16.5°	25.8°
Spatial frequency (cycles/degree)	8.1	8.9	10.3
Score	17/30	20/30	17/30
Spatial frequency (cycles/degree)	5.2	5.7	6.6
Score	15/30	19/30	19/30
Spatial frequency (cycles/degree)	1.0	1.1	1.3
Score	24/60	48/60	48/60
Estimated threshold (cycles/degree)	< 1.0	2.5	2.9

(October 1974)

Table 15   Acuity—right field

	Eccentricity		
	6.25°	16.5°	25.8°
Spatial frequency (cycles/degree)	9.24	10.8	–
Score	29/30	20/30	–
Spatial frequency (cycles/degree)	8.1	8.9	10.3
Score	30/30	28/30	12/30
Spatial frequency (cycles/degree)	–	7.6	8.8
Score	–	30/30	25/30
Spatial frequency (cycles/degree)	5.2	5.7	–
Score	30/30	30/30	–
Estimated threshold (cycles/degree)	> 10.3	10.3	9.2

(October 1974)

plane, the cycles per degrees are calculated separately for each eccentricity, and are shown in Table 14.

Following this series a similar but abbreviated Latin square design was used for the same eccentricities in the *right* (good) field, but with one higher setting of spatial frequency (85 cycles across the whole grating) and one intermediate setting (60 cycles). The equivalent cycles/degree are presented in Table 15.

Finally, the left field measurements were repeated at with the lowest spatial frequency setting, with one group of 30 trials at each eccentricity, going from farthest to nearest.

Results

As can be seen from Table 14, surprisingly in the impaired left half-field the performance was better at a more peripheral eccentricity than the one nearest to the fovea, opposite to expectation and to the results in the good field. At 6.25° eccentricity, acuity was poorer than 1 cycle/degree; indeed, D.B. never performed better than chance at this eccentricity. At 16.5° eccentricity, it was estimated to be approximately 2.5 cycles/degree, and at 25.8° eccentricity it was of the same order of magnitude (2.9 cycles/degree). The acuity of the points tested in the field defect in all cases was inferior, however, to that of equivalent points tested in the intact right field (Table 15).

Verbal commentaries

For all tests carried out in the *scotoma*, D.B. said that he never had any experience in response to the gratings. For example, immediately after having achieved 28 out of 30 correct in one run, he said, 'I was just guessing — no idea how I did.' In the *intact* field, when he performed at chance, at the most extreme eccentricity, he said he was 'just guessing'. When he was performing well, at the least extreme position, he said he was quite confident, and at intermediate levels he said he was 'sometimes guessing'.

Ives apparatus — central 70° (a)

Later in the evening of the next day (October 1974) acuity over a wider range of eccentricities was tested. The apparatus was kept in a fixed position, and on each trial the fixation point was moved in a quasi-random order horizontally around an angled screen such that there was an angular separation between it and the nearest edge of the grating of 9°, 20°, 32.5°, 44.5°, or 56°. The distance to the fixation point was approximately constant. The apparatus was kept at a fixed number of 9 cycles across the grating; in this condition D.B. was slightly farther away than in the preceding condition, namely, 50.8 cm, which meant the grating was 7.13° across, and the spatial frequency was therefore 1.3 cycles per degree). As the ambient level of illumination was lower as dusk approached, the grating as a whole had a slightly higher contrast and was also more distinctive, but the flux value of

Table 16   Acuity

Eccentricity*	9°	20°	32.5°	44.5°	56°
Score	5/12 8/12	4/12 7/12	8/12 8/12	8/12 11/12	11/12 8/12
Totals	13/24 = 54.2%	11/24 = 45.8%	16/24 = 66.7%	19/24 = 79.2%	19/24 = 79.2%

*Stimulus = 1.3 cycles/degree
(October 1974)

the grating itself remained at 2.0 log ft lamberts. Twelve groups of 10 trials each were given, with each eccentricity occurring twice in each group. Thus, a total of 120 trials was given, 24 trials per eccentricity.

The results are shown in Table 16. Again, along the horizontal meridian, it will be seen that D.B. performed better at peripheral loci than at more central loci.

Verbal commentaries

At the three most eccentric locations, D.B. sometimes said that had an 'impression of shimmering' and when he did he reported 'lines'. As he failed to make such a report in the session earlier in the day, (or when the Ives apparatus was used earlier to test acuity (Weiskrantz *et al.* 1974), it is not clear whether he was more sensitive at these more eccentric positions or whether the difference was due to the change in illumination conditions.

Ives apparatus—central 70° (b)

Conditions could be controlled better when he was tested in a similar way four months later in Oxford in a windowless room. The apparatus was kept in a constant position within the Aimark apparatus, at a distance of 34 cm from D.B., and a small target light that served as a fixation point was moved on every trial so as to vary the distance between the nearest edge of the grating and the fixation point to 10°, 30°, 50°, or 70°. The spatial frequency of the grating was kept constant at 0.85 cycles/degree. Half of the trials, in random sequence, were of the grating, and half of a uniform field matched in flux. For the first 40 trials, the ambient overhead fluorescent lights were on, producing a moderately level of illumination (0.6 log ft lamberts on the white room wall). For the second 40 trials, the illumination was reduced by 0.8 log units by using an anglepoise lamp. Under both conditions, a weaker source of projection was used than before, yielding a light value of 1.9 log ft lamberts when the grating field was uniform. After these 80 trials, an addition 40 trials were given with eccentricity held constant at 50°. Finally, later in the session an additional 80 trials were given with a stronger projector source (2.0 log ft lamberts) at six different eccentricities between 15° and 90°.

Results

These are summarized in Table 17. As in previous tests along the horizontal meridian, performance was better at some peripheral eccentricities than nearer the fovea. He performed at 78.3 per cent correct at 50°, but was at chance at more central loci. He also fell to chance at 70°. An independent test of his performance in his good field at 70° under the same conditions yielded a score of 80 per cent (32/40) so as before, his acuity is poorer in the scotoma than in the good field. When the projector source was made stronger, the same general shape of function was found (Table 18), but elevated — his performance at 45° eccentricity reaching 93 per cent (27/29).

Table 17   Acuity

Eccentricity* (uniform field = 1.9 log ft lamberts)	10°	30°	50°	70°
Ambient = 0.6 log ft lamberts	6/10	4/10	7/10	7/10
Ambient = − 0.2 log ft lamberts	4/10	5/10	{ 7/10 33/40	4/10
Totals	10/20	9/20	47/60	11/20

*Stimulus = 0.85 cycles/degree
(February 1975)

Table 18   Acuity

Eccentricity* (uniform field = 2.0 log ft lamberts)	15°	30°	45°	60°	75°	90°
Ambient = − 0.2 log ft lamberts	6/10	7/12	{ 9/9 18/20	7/9	6/10	3/10
Totals	6/10	7/12	27/29	7/9	6/10	3/10

*Stimulus = 0.85 cycles/degree
(February 1975)

Verbal commentaries

No note is entered of his commentaries in this test.

Acuity using photographs of gratings

For a series of tests in February 1975, matt prints were prepared from photographs of vertically oriented sine wave gratings displayed on an oscilloscope (we are grateful to Mr J. Broad for his care in preparing the prints). They were mounted on stiff cards. On any trial a card with a grating or a uniform flux-matched card was mounted at a predetermined eccentricity on the Aimark perimeter arc. A target light at 100° eccentricity to the right provided a constant fixation point. The cards were $17.6° \times 17.6°$. The test was carried out with overhead fluorescent room illumination, which produced a level of 0.6 log ft lamberts on the white background wall of the room behind the perimeter. Spatial frequency was held constant within each group of 20 trials, and the eccentricity varied on a pseudo-random schedule among angles of 10°, 30°, 50°, and 70°, all on the horizontal meridian. Half of the trials contained gratings, and randomly interposed, the other half contained a uniform card matched in flux. D.B. was instructed to respond 'lines' or 'no lines'. Between trials the cards were covered by a masking card which was removed at the beginning of a trial. Contrast was held constant throughout; using SEI photometer readings of a very low spatial frequency card, it was calculated as 78 per cent $[100 \times (peak - trough)//peak + trough)]$. The following spatial frequencies were used, in the following order: 3.2, 2.1, 1.16, 0.69, 0.34, 0.23, 0.69, 1.16, 0.23 cycles/degree. After this series, a single group of 20 trials was given at the most sensitive eccentricity (30°) using a spatial frequency of 0.69 cycles/degree.

Results

Under these conditions, D.B. performed poorly at a macular locus, and better at more peripheral loci. In the present series the best performance was obtained at 30° eccentricity. In the repeat run at the end, using 0.69 cycles/degree, this competence was confirmed by a performance of 85 per cent (17/20). The overall results are summarized in Table 19, which contains the calculated threshold values and the overall performance levels as a function of eccentricity and also of spatial frequency.

Verbal commentaries

There is no note of his commentaries, but under these conditions of relatively high ambient illumination used with the photographs (0.6 log ft

Table 19   Acuity using photos of gratings

I. *Overall performance for all gratings between 0.23 and 2.1 cycles/degree*
Eccentricity n = 40 per location

10°	30°	50°	70°
57.5%	92.5%	77.5%	55%

II. *Approximate thresholds (cycles/degree)*
Eccentricity (horizontal meridian)

10°	30°	50°	70°
0.51	2.65	0.925	<0.23

III. *Overall performance at all eccentricities between 10° and 70°*
Cycles/degree

0.23	0.69	1.16	2.1	3.2
85%	77.5%	60%	65%	40%

(February 1975)

lamberts), it would have been unusual for D.B. to report any 'waves' or 'feelings'. But no record was made on the occasion of the tests with photographs.

Comment

D.B. was capable of detecting gratings, whether generated by the interference apparatus or photographs, and independently of any necessary acknowledged experience. A comparison of three acuity test series with varying eccentricity along the horizontal meridian, with spatial frequency either held constant ('Ives' apparatus) or summed over all spatial frequencies used ('cards'), is plotted in Fig. 23, in which a similar trend is seen in each series, acuity improving with eccentricity out to about 30° to 45°, and then

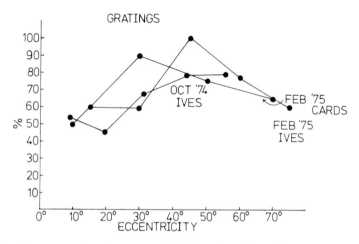

Fig. 23. Summary of performance with detection of grating as a function of eccentricity on the horizontal meridian, showing results for diffraction apparatus (Ives) and photographs of gratings (cards).

declining beyond that region, although the maximum varies with the particular conditions of the test. His acuity is, therefore, measurable, but is clearly reduced in relation to the acuity of his good right half-field. The monkey without striate cortex also shows reduced acuity by approximately 2 octaves (Miller, Pasik, and Pasik 1980) and it is interesting that this is the order of magnitude of reduction for the region 16°–20° eccentric of the impaired field (Table 14) as compared with the intact field (Table 15) when tested under comparable conditions (although the reduction was less than that in our original study, where the conditions were not comparable). At any rate, the results would make any interpretation in terms of stray light artefact difficult to accept, and this point is further bolstered by the fact that his acuity is actually poorer, with both forms of the grating stimuli, close to the vertical meridian than at slightly greater eccentricities.

6 Movement thresholds

While typically D.B. resolutely denied 'seeing' in response to visual stimuli, even though he might sometimes have a 'feeling', we discovered early in our investigations one exception: a very vigorously moving stimulus would elicit a response of genuine 'seeing' in many regions of his field defect. The experience was, however, not veridical: instead of describing a moving stimuli, he spoke instead of complex patterns of radiating lines and grids (see below). Clearly, it was desirable to examine more closely his sensitivity to movement and the conditions under which he would acknowledge 'seeing'.

We examined his capacity informally on a number of occasions with the methods of Riddoch (1917), but to obtain quantitative measures of sensitivity, we used two different set-ups. In the first the amplitude of movement of a spot on an oscilloscope was varied. In the second, a mirror attached to a galvanometer reflected the beam from a projector on to a screen, allowing movement to be generated for any stimulus on a projector slide; the galvanometer was driven by a signal generator (we are very grateful to Mr B. Morton for his help in setting up this experiment). In both arrangements, because we were attempting to simulate the sort of change of intensity involved in clinical testing of the Riddoch type and also because it was not clear over what excursion movement would have to travel in order for it to be detected by D.B., the frequency of oscillation was held constant in any set of determinations and the amplitude of the excursion back and forth was varied to obtain threshold determinations. Hence, velocity and amplitude were confounded. Because the threshold excursions involved turned out to be quite small, typically of the order of 0.25° of visual angle, velocity is likely to have been the primary determinant of sensitivity, but it would be necessary to test this independently as a useful extension.

Movement of oscilloscope point ('shimmer')

In tests carried out in February 1975, a single spot, 3 mm × 3 mm, on an oscilloscope with rapid-decay phosphor was adjusted in brightness to the highest value that did not produce a halo on the screen. It was oscillated sinisoidally up and down at a frequency of 7 Hz. The total distance which the spot traversed could be adjusted by a potentiometer. The screen of the oscilloscope was aligned with the end of the Aimark screen, and a spot on the perimeter provided a fixation spot. The eccentricity of fixation was varied along the horizontal meridian between 10° and 90°, in steps of 10°.

Two levels of ambient illumination were used, the first with the overhead fluorescent room lamps on, providing a light level of the white wall immediately behind the oscilloscope of 0.6 log ft lamberts, and the second a dimmer illustration provided by a desk lamp pointing to the corner of the room, yielding a − 0.2 log ft lamberts level of the wall. The level of the spot itself was not measured, but was approximately 1.0 log ft lamberts in the bright ambient condition. At the beginning of the first session (February 1975), with the overhead lights on, the excursion of the spot was held constant and eccentricity of fixation gradually increased until D.B. reported 'seeing'

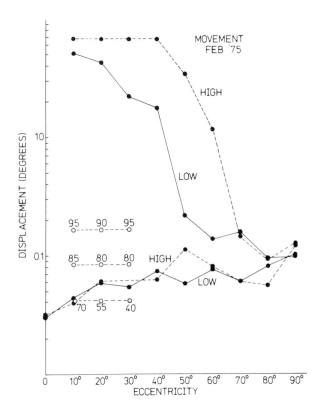

Fig. 24. Results of seen movement of oscillograph spot in impaired left half-field (upper curves) and intact right half-field (lower curves), as a function of eccentricity. 'High' and 'low' refer to two levels of ambient illumination. Dotted horizontal lines in lower left show performance (in per cent correct) at three different field eccentricities for given displacements vs. no displacement when D.B. was forced to guess whether spot was moving or not in his impaired field. Interpolated threshold values of 75% approximate the threshold levels for seen movement in the intact right half-field. (See text for further details)

something in the region of the oscilloscope face. This occurred at about 50° eccentricity. Then the eccentricity was shifted in 10° steps, starting at 90° and working inwards towards the fovea, and then outwards again. At each eccentricity, D.B. was asked to adjust the potentiometer up and down to the weakest setting which just allowed him to detect something on the screen. The same method was also used to determine thresholds in the intact half-field.

The results are shown in Fig. 24. The top two lines are for the defective left half-field, and the bottom two for the intact right half-field, in each case for the two levels of ambient illumination. The thresholds for the impaired field are markedly elevated (note that the ordinate is a log scale), and show a slope opposite to that of the intact field. In fact, with the high level of ambient illumination, it was not possible to obtain a threshold for eccentricities of less than 40° using an excursion over the whole face of the oscilloscope.

Oscilloscope movement threshold by forced-choice 'guessing'

The results just reported for conscious awareness of a moving stimulus showed a clear bias towards peripheral vision along the horizontal meridian. But the question arose as to whether his sensitivity for movement would show a similar pattern if he was tested by forced-choice guessing for excursions that were below threshold for conscious report, i.e., if he were tested in the same way as for other stimulus situations in which he was devoid of any perceptual experience. To test this, groups of 20 trials were given in half of which the spot was actually moving, and in the other half of which it was stationary. Ambient illumination was set at the 'low' level. Three different excursions were used, at eccentricities of 10°, 20°, and 30°, as indicated by the short horizontal lines in the lower left region of Fig. 23. D.B. was required to respond by guessing 'moving' or 'not moving' on each trial.

The results were surprising. The actual percentage correct scores (out of 20) are shown by the numbers entered above the lines in Fig. 24. It will be seen that his sensitivity by guessing was very markedly improved in relation to the thresholds for reported 'seeing'. Indeed, they were of the same general order of magnitude as the 'seeing' thresholds for the good field. That forced-choice thresholds should be somewhat better than method of limits is not unexpected, especially as the former are based on a 75 per cent definition whereas method of limits, when only the ascending direction of stimulus increase is used (as in this specific example), adopts a definition of 100 per cent or close to 100 per cent. With projection method of studying movement (below), we could compare the two psychophysical methods directly for the same stimulus changes and, as will be seen, the method of limits produced a threshold that was about two to three times the value of the forced-choice thresholds. But in the present case there is increase in sensitivity by forced-choice guessing of some sixty-fold! A second surprise was that the slope of the function relating threshold to eccentricity appears to be the same as for the normal field, unlike that of the function of 'seen' stimuli. There was not time to measure points further eccentric, but unless there were to be 'supernormal' in sensitivity, the sign of the slope of the 'guessing' function with eccentricity is very likely to be the same as his normal curve.

Verbal commentaries

For the forced-choice situation just described, D.B. reported having no experience whatever. Immediately after a run in which he performed at 95 per cent correct, he said after questioning, 'I had no feeling of movement. It was all guess-work'. Q: 'Did you have *any* feeling?' A: 'No'.

For those runs in which he was asked to adjust the apparatus until he had an awareness of a visual event, he had difficulty in giving a precise description. It was not, he said, an experience of a moving spot, but more like a curved gridwork of lines. After one run, he drew a cluster of four inverted U-shaped lines, arranged in a nest one immediately above the other, and said that he saw 'egg-shaped lines moving up'. At other times he described 'radiating' lines in a complex arrangement.

Projected moving stimuli

All of this testing was carried out in September 1979 in the light-proof laboratory used in the 'standard situation' (see below). All testing in the scotoma was carried out in the lower left quadrant, and always along the meridian 45° off-horizontal. The background illumination of the test quadrant was − 1.05 log ft lamberts. The other three quadrants were flooded with light from six lantern projectors, two per quadrant, producing an ambient level on each of 0.40 log ft lamberts. A silent, motor-driven mirror was mounted immediately in front of projector (Kodak Carousel, adapted as a projecting tachistoscope, Forth Instruments), enabling us to project any lantern slide onto a screen, which was placed 1 metre in front of the subject. The mirror was driven by a signal generator in which the frequency, amplitude, and wave-form could be varied. The wave-form was always triangular, thus driving the mirror back and forth at a uniform velocity over each traverse.

Two types of moving images were used, both projected along the 45° lower left meridian; they always moved back and forth horizontally: (a) a vertical line, 10° long by 0.5° wide. The line was 0.8 log ft lamberts and hence appeared as a lighter bar on a darker ground; (b) a circular disc of light, 1.84 log ft lamberts, 10° in diameter, projected onto a dark field. The frequency of the triangular wave was always set at one of four settings: 2.45, 5.39, 11.13, or 16.12 Hz. The amplitude of the wave was varied in order to obtain a threshold. This was done in one of two ways. The amplitude of the wave was gradually increased ('method of limits') by the experimenter turning the controlling potentiometer until D.B. responded with a positive verbal response, 'now!' When the method of limits was used, the frequencies were always presented first in ascending order and then in descending order, for at least 4 complete cycles. Or, the amplitude was held constant for a block of trials; blocks varied upwards or downwards according to a modified 'staircase' method (see Chapter 17), the subject being required to make a forced-choice response of either 'moving' or 'not moving'. In many situations, both methods were used to obtain separate threshold estimates.

Results (a) moving vertical line

When the line was placed at an eccentricity of 25°, he gave reliable threshold determinations by the 'method of limits' for all four frequency settings. The results are shown in Table 20. Compared with control subjects for the same stimulus conditions, D.B. is two to three times less sensitive overall (Table 21). The 5.39 Hz frequency gave the most sensitive threshold value and this remained true for D.B. with either threshold method (control subjects are usually relatively flat in this part of the frequency domain, which is the most sensitive part, although their sensitivity may be slightly better at 11.13 Hz). Using this frequency for the same stimulus and location (25° eccentricity) but with the forced-choice staircase method, a threshold of 0.061° excursion was obtained for D.B. (i.e., about 2½ times more sensitive than value with the method of limits).

The same procedures were then followed for the moving line placed at 45° eccentricity, and also at 15° eccentricity. At 45°, D.B. was too insensitive at all frequencies to obtain a threshold measure by either psychophysical

Table 20   Moving vertical line

	Frequency			
	2.45 Hz	5.39 Hz	11.13 Hz	16.12 Hz
25° eccentricity	0.37° ± 0.08°	0.16° ± 0.05°	0.20° ± 0.05°	0.22° ± 0.08°
15° eccentricity	1.36° ± 0.26°	0.48° ± 0.09°	0.51° ± 0.06°	0.64° ± 0.17°

Mean threshold excursions ± S.D.
(September, 1979)

Table 21   Threshold values for two control subjects. Moving vertical line

	Frequency			
	2.45 Hz	5.39 Hz	11.13 Hz	16.12 Hz
Subject LP	0.140°	0.074°	0.076°	0.12°
Subject EG	0.134°	0.072°	0.062°	0.082°

Mean threshold excursions

method. When the line was placed at 15° eccentricity, the threshold values obtained by 'method of limits' are shown in Table 20. Because he appeared to be less sensitive at this eccentricity than at 25°, contrary to the situation for a normal visual field, the threshold measures using method of limits was repeated for 25°, and indeed it was again appreciably better at 25° than 15° eccentricity. But this did not emerge with the staircase method, where both had approximately had the same value, 0.061° and 0.040° respectively, tested with the 5.39 Hz frequency. It will be noted that the staircase method again yielded a somewhat more sensitive value than the method of limits, by a factor of two to three, as anticipated (see above).

Verbal commentaries

With both psychophysical procedures used with the moving vertical line, D.B.'s response to supra-threshold stimuli was similar. 'I did not see the line. There was a kind of pulsation. I did not see the light or anything, but I could *feel* the movement, and I was absolutely sure of it'. At 45° eccentricity (where he was too insensitive to give thresholds), he said it 'was pure guess-work'.

Results (b) Moving disc

Because the vertical line appeared to be too weak a stimulus for the peripheral field, the larger 10° diameter disc was used to plot sensitivity over a wider range of eccentricities. The light value of the disc measured 1.84 log ft lamberts, with the same ambient light conditions as above. It was, in fact, possible to obtain thresholds for all loci, even beyond 60°. All determinations were made only with the 5.39 Hz frequency. The results for eccentricities out to 45° using the forced-choice staircase method are shown in plot M of Fig. 22 (p. 52), which also shows results for D.B.'s good field. (The values in the figure are plotted in terms of velocity, log degrees per second. The corresponding values in terms of excursion of the stimulus in degrees are: 15° eccentricity, 0.158°; 20° eccentricity, 0.12°; 25° eccentricity, 0.057°; 35° eccentricity, 0.086°; and 45° eccentricity, 3.24°.) Threshold values were also obtained for all loci using the 'method of limits', which typically gave rather higher threshold values, again by a factor of between two and three.

An extended series of tests was also carried out at loci far from the good field, at an eccentricity of more than 60° out along the meridian 45° off-horizontal, and a number of control procedures were employed. In addition to the six projectors flooding the 3 non-test quadrants, a projector was also aimed at the region just below the locus being tested, and it also illuminated the floor between the subject and the screen. The forced-choice threshold was determined to be approximately 3.25° (a log velocity of 1.54°/sec). The excursion was then set at well above threshold, approximately 8°. He performed at 26/30 correct. For the remainder of the tests a dark cloth was then placed so as to cover the floor between him and the screen, to reduce any possible reflections from that surface (although none could actually be seen by us). His performance was 10/10 correct. Then, in addition and for the remainder of the tests, his nose was covered with dark face cream and powder to reduce any possible reflections from that surface. He performed at 18/20. Then the amplitude was reduced below threshold for 90 trials to ensure that he would still be below 75 per cent (he was). Then the 8° amplitude value was reintroduced, and he performed at 14/15 correct. Next, without warning or break in a continuous run of trials, the amplitude was switched to a value well below threshold (excursion of 0.60°), and his performance was 6/15 correct. When switched back to the 8° excursion, again without warning or break, he got 10/10 correct.

Next, the bright fluorescent overhead lights were turned on to reduce contrast (ambient level of test quadrant not measured, but estimated from another test condition to be 0.6 to 0.7 log ft lamberts, with the other three quadrants at 0.9 log ft lamberts), and with the same excursion he scored 40/50. Finally, the eccentricity in the field was increased even further, to the maximum locus without going off the screen onto the floor, approximately 80°. With the full overhead lights on, he performed at 36/50. The overhead lights were then turned off (but the masking projectors, as always, remained on) and he performed at 44/50. The last control run of 50 trials was given to check for possible auditory or other extraneous artefacts with the galvanometer still being driven at the same rate and amplitude. Everything was run as in the previous trials, but the light path was blocked so that no stimulus actually appeared (D.B., of course, understood it to be an ordinary run). He performed at 19/50.

Verbal commentaries

When the stimulus was at 35° eccentricity or less, he said, as he had with the moving vertical line, that he 'saw pulsating waves', which he also sometimes described as 'bent'. At 45° and more eccentric positions, he consistently and insistently said that he 'had no sense of anything. There is nothing at all. I am just guessing'. At the most extreme loci he sometimes said that he felt he had done reasonably well, although he 'did not know why'. But when the final run of 50 'blank' trials was run (without his knowledge, of course, that it was a control run), he commented, 'Just guessing. Just like before, except that I do not think I did very well'.

Comment

Thus, while moving visual stimuli, if vigorous enough, produced an experience genuinely acknowledged to be 'seeing', his sensitivity to movement below that threshold was remarkably impressive. When 'seen', the experience was not veridical. Stimuli below threshold for 'seeing', especially if within 30° of the fixation point, were apt to produce an 'awareness' or 'feeling' of which he was very conscious in his everyday life. But still well below that threshold, he could show forced-choice good sensitivity and levels of performance of 90 per cent to 100 per cent, despite acknowledging no awareness or experience of the stimulus.

7 Discrimination of orientation

Discrimination of orientation of single bars

In our original paper we reported a demonstration of good discrimination of the orientation of successively presented bars, either horizontal vs. vertical or vertical vs. diagonal. We followed this up in a further study in February 1976, when we were also interested in the difference in performance between the left and right eyes (see Chapter 4). The first test, however, was binocular. D.B. was seated in a semi-darkened hospital office room, and a white bar was projected onto the wall for 125 msec. (using a Compar shutter placed in front of a Leitz Type 31 044 000, 150-watt projector). He was told that a vertical or horizontal bar would be flashed into his blind field, and he was to respond either 'up-and-down' or 'across'. The order of each block of 30 trials was quasi-random, and the same slide was used for both orientations. The size of the bar was 21.6 cm long × 1.27 cm wide, and the fixation distance was 91.4 cm. Given their positions in the field, the dimension of the bar in units of visual angle was slightly different in its vertical and horizontal orientations, 26.0° and 23.4° respectively. The vertical bar was 14° to the left of the fixation, and its top edge 4.8° below. The horizontal bar was 16.3° below the fixation and its right edge 14° to the left. D.B. performed at 80 per cent correct (48/60). Because we had found that discrimination was a function of size of stimulus, we also used a larger stimulus (94.0 cm long × 1.3 cm wide. The vertical bar was 32.9° to the left of the fixation point, with its top edge 9.6° below; the horizontal bar was 17.2° below the fixation point, with its right edge 22.9° to the left). He performed better, but only marginally so, at 83.3 per cent (25/30).

Later in the session we compared with two eyes on a horizontal vs. vertical discrimination. The ambient illumination was not measured, but was provided by an anglepoise lamp in the corner of the room and hence was moderately dim. The contrast of the projected stimuli was light upon dark ground. The bar was 48.3 cm long when in the vertical orientation and 47.0 cm in the horizontal orientation. The vertical bar was 23.8° to the left of the fixation point, with its top edge 5.0° below. The horizontal bar was 17.9° below the fixation point, with its right edge 13.2° to the left. Blocks of 30 trials were presented, in the order LRRL eye. There was a gradual trend towards improvement as the experiment proceeded: the two left eyes scores were 21/30 and 28/30 = 81.7% overall; the right eye scores were 17/30 and 25/30 = 70% overall. Thus, as in the 'presence vs. absence' detection series, the scores of the left eye were somewhat superior to those of the right.

Verbal commentaries

He was questioned very closely about his response to horizontal and vertical orientations separately. He was insistent that he had no experience of either. 'Not aware of anything'; 'There is nothing to guide me'. With the short lines (80% correct) he said he was not confident, and judged that he was performing at chance. When the lines were lengthened, he said that he was 'not aware of anything, but I am pretty confident'. His comments during the monocular experiments were similar: 'I did not get anything to go on'; 'Pure guess-work' (this immediately after performing 28/30 correct). On one occasion with his right eye, he said very tentatively 'Maybe there was a little shadow — not sure'. Throughout he was 'not confident' about how well he had performed.

Orientation of a grating in a circular aperture

While the results with single bars were clear, the situation is obviously confounded by the inherent necessity for the alternative stimuli to occupy different positions in the visual field. We have already seen that the equi-eccentric positions in the field cannot be assumed to be uniform either in their sensitivity or acuity. An arrangement that circumvents this difficulty is a grating, 50 per cent dark-light, placed in a circular aperture within which the orientation of the grating can be varied.

The grating we used was, in all cases, in a circular aperture 10° in diameter. It was projected onto a tangent screen by a projecting tachistoscope with a zoom lens that allowed the size to be adjusted so that was the angular size kept constant at different retinal eccentricities. The environment was always that of the 'standard situation', with two projectors flooding each of three quadrants not being tested. The test quadrant was the lower left, with a background illumination of − 1.05 log ft lamberts. The level of the three illuminated quadrants outside the testing quadrant was 0.40 log ft lamberts. The grating was square wave, 0.9 cycles per degree. The duration was always 150 msec. The light bars in the grating had a photometer reading of 0.80 log ft lamberts, the dark 0.00 log ft lamberts.

In April 1982 we measured his orientation discrimination sensitivity along the 45° off-horizontal meridian at the following eccentricities: 45°, 35°, 25°, and 15°. Thresholds were determined using the modified staircase procedure (see Chapter 17). One of the two orientations was always horizontal, the other non-horizontal, and D.B. was asked always to respond 'across' or 'not across'. The initial setting was with the non-horizontal orientation at 90°

i.e. vertical. The staircase steps were 45°, 35°, 25°, 15° and 10° off-horizontal vs. horizontal. The results are shown in Fig. 22 (p. 52), graph O, which also shows comparative results for the lower right (intact) quadrant. (In this case, of course, the background projectors were changed so as to illuminate the lower left quadrant instead of the lower right, and an additional 5° step was added to the series. As this was the smallest orientation difference available, all that can be said about the narrowest eccentricity, 15°, in the good field is that the difference threshold must be less than 5°). It will be seen that at 45° eccentricity in the scotoma he was unable to discriminate even horizontal vs. vertical (17/30 correct), but at the next smaller eccentricity he was able to achieve the highly creditable threshold of 12.81° difference in orientation, and thereafter he remained quite good, although his sensitivity was, in fact, better at 35° eccentricity than it was closer to the fovea. His sensitivity was always worse than in his good field, but by no less than a factor of about two at 35° eccentricity.

One brief experiment was also run in 1982 comparing the two eyes, both for the same eccentricity: 25° on the 45° off-horizontal meridian in the lower left quadrant. The lighting conditions were identical to those just described. He was given blocks of 10 trials with a horizontal vs. a vertical grating in the order left–right–right–left eyes. He was too close to ceiling for the results to be illuminating, although there was a tendency for the right eye, as in other tests, to be inferior. With the left eye he achieved 100 per cent (20/20), and with the right eye, 90 per cent (19/20).

When tested in 1983, some parts of D.B.'s field had become 'lively', and in one procedure we deliberately tried to arrange conditions to reduce the potentially distracting or supporting effect of the 'waves' which had started to become a common feature of his reports (see Chapter 13). The same procedure was adopted as with squares vs. diamonds and squares vs. rectangles in Chapter 8). The level of ambient illumination was increased from −1.05 to 0.60 log ft lamberts on the test quadrant in the 'standard situation'. This was achieved by using bright overhead fluorescent room lamps, together with the flooding projectors which illuminated the other three quadrants, producing on them an ambient level of 0.95 log ft lamberts. The standard grating was used for orientation testing, i.e., 0.9 cycles/degree in a circular aperture of 10° diameter. The level of the light bar in the grating was 0.90 log ft lamberts, and of the dark bar, 0.68 log ft lamberts. The testing was carried out with the centre of the grating at an eccentricity of 45° along the lower 45° meridian, which under these conditions was quite 'dead'. Runs of 20 trials each were given for horizontal grating vs. grating orientations of 15°, 15°, 10°, 5°, 20°, and 45°, in that order. As before, he had to respond 'across' or 'not across'. The results, arranged in decreasing order of orientation difference, were: 45°: 19/20; 20°: 17/20; 15°: 33/40; 10°: 15/20; 5°: 13/20. Thus, his threshold value (75%) is 10°, which is superior to any level of performance he had previously shown at this eccentricity, even though contrast was substantially lower in the present case. The results are discussed in more detail in Chapter 13.

Verbal commentaries

These showed an interesting dissociation between performance and acknowledged experience. At 45° eccentricity in the first high contrast condition, where he was still at chance, perhaps not surprisingly he said it was 'pure guess-work'. But at 35°, where he had a threshold as small as 12.8° orientation difference, he made precisely the same comment: 'Pure guess-work. I do not even have any idea of a flash'. This was true even for the most extreme difference, horizontal vs. vertical, where of course he achieved 90 per cent performance. At 25° eccentricity he said that he had an impression of 'something coming in' when the stimuli was flashed on, but he 'was guessing about *orientation*'. Later, in the final ascending portion of the staircase, when he reached 19/20, he said, 'I *think* I say "across" when the bolt coming out is thinner, and "not-across" when it is thicker. But maybe not. It is somewhat like what my moving finger looks like when I close my eyes, in my imagination'. Finally, with the narrowest eccentricity, he said, 'one is definitely thicker than the other — I say "across" when it is thin, but I don't know whether I am right or not'. In the brief experiment comparing the two eyes, he said 'I think I did better with my left eye than my right eye. There was more a definite movement when I said "across" than when I said "up and down". Not so much movement with my right eye'.

It may be noted that under the first high contrast condition his sensitivity at 15° and 25° eccentricity, where he had an experience of something occurring, was actually slightly poorer than at 35° eccentricity, where he said that he did not have any idea even of the on/off of the stimulus field itself and where he was insistent that his performance was based on pure guess-work.

This was even more striking under the low contrast conditions intended to abolish the distracting waves in the 1983 tests, when his performance was better at 45° eccentricity than it had ever been previously, and where he achieved an orientation difference threshold of 10°. Under these conditions deliberately arranged to abolish any subjective response, he said 'Nothing at all. Not even a sense of a flash'; 'Just guessing'; 'Not a hint of anything'. After getting 95 per cent (19/20) correct for horizontal vs. 45°, he said, 'Nothing at all'; 'Just 50/50, did not do very well'. This type of comment was recorded after every run in the series.

Comment

Among the residual capacities demonstrated in D.B., orientation must be reckoned to be one of the most sensitive. Although still impaired relative to the good field, a discrimination of a difference of 10° for an eccentricity of 45° from fixation is highly creditable and, in fact, was exactly the same as the threshold in the good field at this eccentricity obtained a year previously (but under different contrast conditions). As with other discriminations, under certain conditions he had some type of experience (non-veridical), but the impressive outcome was that his performance actually was superior when conditions were arranged to abolish any acknowledged experience whatever, even of the flash of the onset of the grating field.

8   'Form' discrimination

We studied D.B.'s ability to discriminate shapes, using various letters, rectangles vs. squares, and degrees of curvature of triangles. In most studies we used both projected and back-illuminated material.

X vs. O

The letter discrimination most often used was **X** vs. **O**, as this had already been examined in our first study (with projected stimuli) and revealed a good capacity, especially when the letters were of large size.

Back-illuminated letters

In October 1974 and February 1975 we used an alternative to projected stimuli. In effect, the arrangement was equivalent to a 'light box'. Glass plates were inserted behind the aperture of the Ives acuity apparatus (see above), allowing them to be illuminated from behind. The diffusing plate of the apparatus was between the lamp (60 watts) and the glass plate. Opaque figures either of black Letraset or shaped from black plastic tape were mounted on the glass plates, giving the appearance of a solid black letter on a diffusely lit white ground. The light level of the white ground was 2.0 log ft lamberts, and of the black figure 1.1 log ft lamberts. The entire apparatus was in front of a white wall which had a photometer level of − 0.2 log ft lamberts. The fixation distance was 37 cm and the centre of each stimulus was 20° eccentric from the fixation point along the horizontal meridian in the left field. **X**s and **O**s were formed, in this experiment, from Letraset material (sheets 709A and B). The size of the **X** was 6.5° × 5.4°, and the **O** was 6.6° × 5.9°, each with a thickness of approximately 1.2°. Two blocks of 20 trials each were given. D.B. scored 18 and 19 correct in each, respectively, or 92.5 per cent overall. The stimuli used here were somewhat smaller than those which yielded comparable performance levels with projected stimuli at an earlier phase of testing (Weiskrantz *et al.* 1974).

Projected stimuli

In February 1976 we repeated the same type of projection procedure as had been used originally. Slides of **X**s and **O**s were prepared of various sizes and positions in the field, and also the contrast (i.e., black on white, white on black). In this series, the duration was 125 msec. Each stimulus was presented singly, and D.B. asked to respond '**X**' or '**O**'. Nine blocks of 30 trials each were given. The stimulus conditions, in the order in which the tests were carried out, and results are summarized in Table 22. (The thickness of the letters throughout was 2° to 2.4°). The level of ambient light on the screen during the first and last five conditions was not measured, but was relatively dim, provided by a desk lamp at some 6 feet or so from the light coloured wall on which the stimuli were projected. During the remaining three blocks, the bright fluorescent overhead lights were also turned on, which yielded a high level of ambient illumination on the projections screen and low contrast for the stimuli. It will be seen that in all cases but one, D.B. was above chance. The difference between the condition yielding chance performance and all others is that in the former case the stimuli fell farther eccentrically, and were also relatively small (but not the smallest) among the set as a whole. It will be noted that when the contrast is 'black on white' any effect of stray light would be inverted, i.e., it is the background rather than the stimulus that may be intruding into the good field.

Table 22   **X** vs. **O** discriminations

Stimulus		Height	Width	Contrast	Nearest point to fixation (degrees)	Meridian (below horizontal) of nearest point	Performance
1	X	9.2°	6.8°	W on B	16.0°	39.9°	22/30
	O	10.1°	8.7°		16.0°	39.9°	
2	X	14.9°	11.1°	W on B	19.9°	29.1°	27/30
	O	16.2°	13.6°		19.9°	29.1°	
3	X	13.8°	10.5°	B on W	23.6°	42.4°	26/30
	O	15.0°	13.4°		17.8°	40.8°	
4	X	13.0°	9.9°	W on B	24.0°	43.8°	30/30
	O	14.4°	12.9°		19.4°	45.0°	
5	X	12.4°	9.3°	W on B	29.8°	32.9°	22/30
	O	14.7°	11.4°		25.2°	28.1°	
6	X	12.5°	8.7°	W on B	34.0°	37.9°	11/30
	O	14.2°	11.6°		29.1°	38.6°	
7	X	16.5°	11.3°	W on B	17.8°	26.6°	25/30
	O	16.5°	13.2°		17.8°	26.6°	
8	X	14.7°	9.6°	W on B	25.8°	16.8°	23/30
	O	15.7°	11.2°		25.8°	16.8°	
9	X	14.7°	9.6°	W on B	25.8°	16.8°	25/30
	O	15.7°	11.2°		25.8°	16.8°	

(February, 1976)

In April 1977 we again repeated the same procedure, except that the duration was 100 msec and the illumination conditions were different. All conditions were 'black on white'. In the first block of 30 trials, the **X** was $13.6° \times 9.6°$, the top edge $5.7°$ below the fixation and the right edge $16.7°$ to its left. The **O** was $14° \times 11.7°$, the top edge $5.7°$ below the fixation and the right edge $14.9°$ to its left. The thickness of the letters was $2.6°$. During the first 10 trials (when he performed 9/10), with the room illumination relatively dim, he complained that there was too much glare from the projected background of the stimulus, and so the overhead lights were turned on and the intensity of the projector reduced. The ambient level on the screen at that point and thereafter was 1.25 log units. The level of the white background during the stimulus presentation was 1.95 log ft lamberts, and of the **X** and **O** was 1.45 log ft lamberts. During these remaining 20 trials, he again made only one error. Then, without changing the lighting conditions, we reduced the size of the stimuli (**X** $= 4.4° \times 3.3°$, top $5.7°$ below fixation, right edge $20.1°$ to its left. **O** $= 6.1° \times 4.8°$, top $5.7°$ below fixation, right edge $17.8°$ to its left. The thickness was $0.7°$ to $0.9°$). His performance was perfect, 30/30. Finally, we reduced the size still further (**X** $= 1.4° \times 0.9°$, top $5.7°$ below fixation, right edge $11.3°$ to its left. **O** $= 2.2° \times 1.8°$, top $5.2°$ below fixation, right edge $10.4°$ to its left, thickness $0.3°$). His performance then fell to 10/30 correct. Thus, as in our original study, discrimination depends upon the stimuli being larger than a minimal size, although under the present conditions he could do somewhat better with small stimuli than he could under the conditions of the original study (where his size threshold for **X** vs. **O** appeared to be about $10°$, and in the present experiments between $5°$ and $2°$). Again, 'black on white', despite the inversion of the stray light, yielded good levels of performance.

The **X** vs. **O** discrimination was also studied at some length in a situation in which we compared his ability to match stimuli in the impaired with the good field and within the impaired field; the results are reported below in Chapters 14 and 15.

Verbal commentaries

During the back-illuminated letters trial (February 1975), despite his excellent performance of 92.5 per cent over 40 trials, D.B. reported that 'it was 100 per cent guess-work. I was not aware of anything'.

The situation was somewhat more complex with the projected stimuli. For the white-on-black contrast condition (first two rows, Table 22) he claimed 'I just guessed for **X** and **O**. There was nothing to guide my judgment. Q: Any feeling? A: No, nothing at all'. But for three of the remaining blocks, he did report some experience of the stimuli. Thus, after Row 3 condition, he said, sometimes there was 'a smooth, dark and clear "shape". I didn't *see* it — it was just shades darker than the surround. If it wasn't there I said "X"'. After the Row 4 condition, he said there is 'a darkness in the shape of a half letter J. Then I say, "**O**". I say "**X**" when I don't get that feeling'. And, finally, after the Row 7 condition, he said, 'I think I am getting a shadow coming in or out. I am pretty confident. Going one way I say "**X**", going other way, I say "**O**"'. But in the other conditions in which he still performed above chance, i.e., Rows 5, 8, and 9 (as well as the one condition in which he did not, Row 6), he insisted that he was 'simply guessing'. After the last condition (Row 9), when he made 5 errors out of 30 trials, he said, 'Not sure of anything—no shadows. There was nothing to go on'.

In the one condition where he was performing at chance (and in which he said he was guessing), the stimuli were the most eccentrically placed of all those in the set, and they were also relatively small. The condition in which he reported some experience were when the positions of the stimuli were of relatively central eccentricity and largish sizes. Large size appeared to be insufficient to account for the pattern of results without also taking eccentricity into account, because the stimuli for Row 9 were of the same order of size as those of Rows 3 and 4. Therefore, it seems that stimuli near the fixation point (but still more than 15° away from it) were more likely to generate an experience than stimuli some 10° farther away. But even stimuli as close as 16° to 20° from the fixation (Rows 1 and 2) did not generate any experience under the conditions of those blocks. But the contrast conditions there were different, and in Row 1 the stimuli were also relatively small in relation to the others in the set. As regards the contrast, it may be noted the stimuli in blocks 2 and 3, which had opposite contrast conditions, were comparable in size and eccentricity, and so were his levels of performance. In block 3, with black on white, where the stray light situation is inverted, he reported 'a shadowy something'. In block 2, with white on black, where there is a greater problem over a possible stray light artefact, he reported 'just guessing; nothing to guide me'. Why this difference in reported experience should have occurred is unclear, but it speaks against stray light itself as being important.

Finally, with the series in February 1976 and April 1977, in which the size of projected stimuli was progressively reduced, D.B. reported an experience of 'roughness' and 'smoothness' in those blocks of trials in which he performed well. 'Q: Did you see? A: No, but I was sure'. With the smallest size, when he fell to chance, he said he 'was just guessing, although I was aware there was something there'. All of the eccentricities (to the nearest point of the stimuli) in which there was a reported experience in this series were relatively narrow (between 15° and 21°, along meridia between 15° and 21° below-horizontal), which is consistent with the findings above. In so far as one can hazard a summary, it would appear that nearness to the fixation point (for these meridia) plus largish size both favour above chance performance, and that if the stimuli are large enough or near enough they are more likely to be accompanied by an experience, although the experience need not be veridical (e.g., 'moving in' or 'moving out'). It is also the case that good performance can be obtained with his firm denial of any experience or stratagem other than 'guessing'.

Other alpha-numeric discriminations

In February 1975, we also tested a discrimination between a **T** and a **4** by mounting Letraset figures (Sheets 709A and B) on glass plates and back-illuminating the plates in the Ives apparatus, as in the previous arrangement (see above) and with the same lighting conditions. The distance from the stimuli to the subject was 37 cm and the midlines of the stimuli were 20° eccentric from the fixation point along the horizontal meridian. The size of each figure was $6.2° \times 4.9°$. D.B. was first shown the two figures, and then in formal testing was required to make a forced-choice response between them. In 20 trials he made five errors = 75 per cent correct. While a creditable performance, it is still poorer than in the good field, where he was marginally better with the same stimuli at the much greater eccentricity of 70°.

A series of discriminations among five letters (**A, C, D, R,** and **S**) was also tested, using the same back-illuminated arrangement, but at 50° eccentricity. The stimuli were black Letraset from the same series as above (Sheets 709A and B). He was told that the stimulus would also be one of the five letters, and was shown them before the test. In formal testing, each stimulus presentation was 2 seconds. D.B. performed at 17/40 correct; a chance score would be 8/40. While this is a creditable result for such a wide eccentricity, nevertheless in his good field he performed better (26/40) on the same task, at an even wider eccentricity of 70°.

Verbal commentaries

No commentary was recorded for either of these runs. But as the **T** vs. **4** condition immediately followed the back-illuminated **X** vs. **O** discrimination, in which he performed better and about which he insisted that it was '100 per cent guess-work', we may assume that he would have reported any change in his experience in the new task, which was carried out under identical conditions and with stimuli of the same size.

Triangle vs. X

Using the same back-illumination conditions as above, in October 1974 we tested D.B. on a discrimination between a triangle and an **X**, both shaped from black plastic insulating tape. The **X** was $7.7° \times 7.7°$, and the triangle 7.7° along each side. The thickness of the tape was 1.9°. The stimuli were 18.2° eccentric from fixation, on the horizontal meridian. The tests formed part of a larger series concerned with 'double dissociation' between form and detection (see below), but we report this portion here because it is noteworthy that D.B. performed so poorly. In two blocks of 30 trials, his score was 14 and 15 correct, a chance result, despite the slightly larger size of these stimuli and their slightly narrower eccentricity than the **X** vs. **O** task, on which he performed at better than 90 per cent (see above). In another section we discuss the question of whether for D.B. some 'form' discriminations may have their basis in an orientation discrimination, and the present findings may have a bearing on that issue.

Verbal commentary

Perhaps not surprisingly, given his chance performance, D.B. said this task 'was all guess-work'.

Curved vs. straight outline triangles

This discrimination forms part of the 'standard situation' procedure, in which a threshold for curvature is determined for one fixed position in the field. Discussion of results in that situation can be found in Chapter 17. It was also used in one of the tests of 'double dissociation', and those results will be discussed in Chapter 16. In the tests described here, the stimuli consisted of photographs of high contrast black outline drawings, on white grounds, of equilateral triangles whose sides were either straight (the standard) or were curved. The prints were mounted on stiff cardboard. A series of seven degrees of curvature was constructed, from C-7 (most curved) to C-1. Each series was prepared in three different sizes. The smallest set had sides 10.2 cm long (i.e., 16° in the perimeter), and the largest 18.2 cm long (= 28°). The dimensions of the intermediate set were, unfortunately, not recorded, but as it happens that turns out to be unimportant. Illustrations of the actual curvatures are shown in Fig. 25. (We are grateful to Miss Julia Hornak for assistance in preparing the material).

D.B. was first tested with this material in September 1975, at 30°, 45°, and 60° eccentricities. Each stimulus card was attached to the Aimark perimeter by a clip, and covered by a masking card, which was removed to

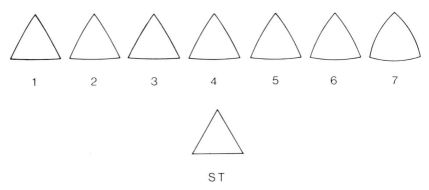

Fig. 25.   Curved outline triangle series.

present the stimulus (for a duration of 2 sec). Blocks of 30 trials were given, always with the straight card as one of the stimuli and a constant degree of curvature as the alternative. The light reading of the white prints was 0.60 log ft lamberts. The intermediate size of stimuli were used. At 60° eccentricity and with the most curved alternative (C-7), he performed at chance (13/30). Similarly, at 30° eccentricity, he was at chance (16/30). But at 45°, he oscillated between chance and 80 per cent correct with the most curved stimulus. In the first two runs with this value he achieved 19/30 and 22/30 = 41/60. The next time he was given this value he did somewhat better, 24/30. With the next least curved stimulus (C-6) his score was 35/60. He was then given the largest stimulus cards for C-7 vs. the straight triangle, and got 20/30. Back to the original size, again, he performed only at 18/30, and finally with a small set of stimuli, C-7 vs. straight (10.2 cm per side), he was at chance, 17/30.

Thus, only in one series did he perform at better than 75 per cent even with the most curved alternative, and it is reasonable to conclude that this discrimination was below his threshold, at least at eccentricities from 30° out to 60°. (In contrast, in his good field at 45° eccentricity, he performed perfectly even with the most difficult discrimination in the smallest sizes series, C-1 vs. straight). We also tried to improve his performance in the impaired field by making the stimuli 'shimmer', on the assumption that this might make them more salient. He performed at marginally above chance, 39/60 = 65 per cent, but still below a threshold value.

In April 1977, we thought it would be worth trying the same discrimination at a more distant eccentricity along the 30° off-horizontal meridian (because there was some evidence that his presence/absence sensitivity was better out there). The stimulus cards were held in position at 74° eccentricity, covered as before with a masking card except when presented for discrimination. The light level on the remainder of the perimeter arc was − 0.9 log ft lamberts, and the white card, itself gave a reading of 0 log ft lamberts. D.B. was given 10 practice trials, plus a run of 30 trials of the easiest discrimination, C-7 vs. standard. He performed at 4/10 + 18/30 = 22/40. (In contrast, in his good field at 78° eccentricity, he achieved 7/10 + 28/30 = 35/40). And so no further evidence could be gathered that he was able to make this discrimination.

Finally, in April 1982, using the set-up in the room for the 'standard situation', he was tested in addition to the easiest discrimination (C-7 vs. straight) with projected stimuli, but at 45° eccentricity on the lower left 45° meridian. The duration of the stimulus was 150 msec. The size of the triangles was increased to the maximum possible setting of the zoom lens, with each side of the straight triangle having an average length of 12.2°. The other three quadrants were flooded by projector lights (see Chapter 17 for light levels as well as his results with the standard triangle discrimination at 25° eccentricity). In 30 trials, he performed at chance, 15/30.

Verbal commentaries

Despite his weak performance in the series with photographic stimulus cards tested at 45° eccentricity, he reported an experience that is difficult to interpret because of its lack of veridicality. With the stationary stimuli, he said he could not detect triangles, but 'it's a circle inside a square — that's the feeling I get'. Making the stimuli shimmer led to no experience at all: 'Not aware of anything. I think I got 50:50 — half right, half wrong'. In the second series at the wider eccentricity, he said he 'was aware of the card [the masking card] being taken away and the area then being clear — if anything, I get a square sort of shape'. Perhaps his report of a 'square' at the earlier stage also derived from the removal of the masking card at the beginning of the trial. Finally, in the series with the projected stimuli in 1982, he reported that 'it was pure guessing. There was no sense of movement'.

April 1982. Square vs. rectangles (a)

There were two reasons for including this series of discriminations. First, Efron (1968) has reported a patient with a severe deficit in this type of discrimination even though acuity was reported as being normal. We have also seen a very similar patient (Warrington 1985) with bilateral inferior occipital damage. If the capacity to discriminate or identify forms is differentially impaired in D.B. (as assessed by objective performance measures, independently of whether he reports any experience or not) as compared with detection, reaching, and other non-form dimensions, it would seem useful to try this type of task. Second, as D.B. can perform orientation discriminations reasonably well, an ambiguity arises in the interpretation of the results of those form discriminations in which the discriminative stimuli had sub-components with different orientations, as for example in **X** vs. **O**. The question is whether the discrimination was between shapes or between orientations. The present shapes avoid that ambiguity.

The first test series was carried out in April 1982. The squares and rectangles were solid, filled, black shapes drawn on white cards 12.5 × 20.5 cm. The black square was 5 cm long (8° 20′) on each side. The series of rectangles were of equal area to the square, and were graded in difficulty. The ratios of width to length, dimensions, going from easiest to most difficult, were as follows:

G:	0.09
F:	0.16
E:	0.36
D:	0.49
C:	0.62
B:	0.82
A:	1.0 (square)

The stimuli were first placed at an eccentricity of 30°, suspended on the arc of the Aimark perimeter, on the lower left 45° meridian. He was given the series in the order **A** vs. **E**, **A** vs. **D**, **A** vs. **C**, **A** vs. **D**, **A** vs. **E** (Fig. 26 shows **A**, **D**, and **E**). For each he had 20 trials in which the square and rectangle were randomly presented in succession for 2 second durations. He was asked to close his eyes between trials while the stimuli were being placed in position. The overhead fluorescent lamps were on, giving a light value on the white of the cards of 1.0 log ft lamberts and on the black of 0.3 log ft lamberts. On each trial he was asked to respond 'square' or 'rectangle'.

Fig. 26. The square and two of the rectangles matched in flux, used in square vs. rectangle series. Middle rectangle (**D**) has ratio of height to length of 0.49; right rectangle (**E**) a ratio of 0.36. (From Weiskrantz and Warrington, in press, by permission).

The results were that he performed well on **A** vs. **E** (18/20 and 17/20 = 87.5%), relatively poorly on **A** vs. **C** (12/20 and 14/20 = 65), and at an intermediate level on the task of intermediate difficulty, **A** vs. **D** (14/20 and 15/20 = 72%). (**A** vs. **C** is still well within the capacity of normal subjects at this eccentricity, although D.B.'s good field was not, in fact, tested). Fig. 26 shows rectangle **D**, which is roughly of threshold value for D.B..

Next, the eccentricity was shifted to 45° (also on the same meridian), and he was given **A** vs. **G**, an easier value than any had been used above. He performed at chance, 11/20. Again, this is well within the limits of control subjects at this eccentricity.

Verbal commentaries

With the stimuli at 30° eccentricity, he said at the beginning of the series and almost until the end, 'there is a lot of movement when I open my eyes, but it is pure guess-work about the shapes'. In the very last block, with **A** vs. **E**, he said 'there are two different movements—one long and the other not so long. I say "rectangle" for the long set of waves'. At that point he thought he did 'above average'. Finally, at the eccentricity of 45°, he said, '50:50 (i.e., chance). There is no movement'.

It is possible that good levels of discrimination between forms for which orientation is not a good differential cue (such as the present ones, curved vs. straight triangles, **X** vs. triangle) may only be possible when the stimuli generate some sort of experience (such as 'movement' or 'sets of waves', not necessarily veridical, in response to the stimulus). This possibility was tested in a further set of experiments. (See also Chapter 13.)

August 1983. Square vs. rectangles (b), and square vs. diamond

The previous results, while supporting the view that 'form' discrimination may actually be derived from orientation discrimination, used a procedure that was far from ideal. The stimulus cards had to be fixed by hand on the perimeter, duration could not be rigidly controlled, and D.B. had to close his eyes between trials, with the attendant difficulty in ensuring good fixation upon opening them. Also, he reported different lengths of 'moving waves' which might have provided a basis for discrimination. In August 1983, we used projected stimuli of the square/rectangle series with a duration of 150 msec. If D.B. is sensitive to orientation rather than 'form', he should perform well on square vs. diamond, which differ only in orientation (45°), and poorly on square vs. rectangles. Finally, in 1983, when the 'wave' phenomena had become generally more intrusive (see Chapter 13), conditions were arranged to abolish them during the discrimination tasks.

Method

Various preliminary arrangements were attempted in order to eliminate the 'waves', which also suggested that when 'waves' were present D.B. attempted to use them. We first tried square vs. diamond (actual size 19.05 cm × 19.05 cm, which equals 8° × 8°) at an eccentricity of 28° on the lower 45° meridian. The light values were −1.12 log ft lamberts for the background in the test quadrant, 1.84 log ft lamberts for the stimulus. He scored 10/10, and reported 'straight line movement'. Exactly the same result and the same experience occurred at 35° eccentricity. Then he was tested at a 40° eccentricity, and his performance fell to 12/20, and he said 'no movement; just guessing'.

A square vs. rectangle series at 35° was then presented, under the same lighting conditions, with results that were curiously irregular. He still had an impression of lines — 'something there, but not seeing anything'. We then reduced contrast of the stimuli with a neutral density filter in the projector path, yielding a stimulus value of 0.2 ft log lamberts on the same background, but with slightly larger stimuli in absolute dimensions (= 7.66° × 7.66°), at the 40° eccentricity, he reported 'something there, but not so much movement'. His performance on square vs. diamond was perfect — 40/40, and he did well with an extreme difference between square and rectangle (**A** vs. **E**, see below), 35/40, but poorly on **A** vs. **D** and **A** vs. **C** (13/20 and 9/20 respectively).

Finally, contrast was reduced severely by turning on full overhead fluorescent lamps, in addition to retaining the flooding projectors in all quadrants except the lower left test quadrant. This, at last, abolished the 'waves'. Under these conditions, the light level on the test quadrant was 0.60 log ft lamberts, and 0.95 on the other three quadrants. The stimuli were 0.9 log ft lamberts. Stimulus exposure was 150 msec. The square and diamond were 7.3° × 7.3° at an eccentricity of 45° on the lower left 45° meridian. The slide series of the rectangles had exactly the same ratios of width to length as the card series above, and are identified by the same letters.

Results and verbal commentaries of 'wave-inhibiting' experiments

As a preliminary check, 40 trials of **X** vs. **O** were given (vertical extent of 10°) at an eccentricity of 45° (on the lower left 45° meridian), for which he scored 32/40. He reported 'nothing there. All guess-work'. This remained true throughout the whole series, during which he was closely questioned after each run. Square (**A**) vs. diamond and **A** vs. rectangle **E** were tested in an ABBA design, 20 trials per run, at the same eccentricity (45°). As mentioned above, the overhead lights were kept on throughout this series.

The result was that he performed at almost 90 per cent for **A** vs. diamond (35/40), and 24/40 for **A** vs. **E**.

By shifting the stimuli to a smaller eccentricity of 35° along the same meridian, the waves returned, and he now succeeded at **A** vs. **D** (39/40) as well as **A** vs. **E** (18/20). On **A** vs. **C**, he dropped to 26/40.

Testing then returned to the wider eccentricity of 45° in order to abolish the waves, and he was tested in runs of 20 trials on **A** vs. **E**, **A** vs. **D**, **A** vs. diamond, **A** vs. diamond, **A** vs. **D**. His scores were excellent on **A** vs. diamond (38/40). On **A** vs. **E** he now showed an improved performance over his previous test, 17/20. On **A** vs. **D**, his score was 28/40. Again he reported no experience at all, whether or not he was performing well. After each run he said, 'nothing at all' 'Guess-work' 'Not even a sense of a flash' 'Did 50:50'.

Although D.B.'s intact right half-field was not tested, the value on which he breaks down in his left half-field is well within the capacity of control subjects tested under comparable conditions of contrast (difference of 0.3 log ft lamberts), 150 msec duration, at 45° eccentricity on the lower 45° meridian). On **A** vs. **D**, three control subjects made perfect scores, and on **A** vs. **C**, they scored a mean of 90 per cent. On **A** vs. **B**, two control subjects scored 17/20 and 18/20 correct.

A summary of all those 'form' and grating orientation tests for which D.B. reported having no subjective experience is contained in Tables 23–26.

Comment

Thus, when orientation was the only cue D.B.'s performance was excellent under these conditions, and in the absence of any subjective experience. When 'shape' was degraded, with orientation held constant, his performance was also degraded, although if the difference in length was great enough he could succeed. Of course, as length increases and width decreases, the rectangle itself assumes an increasingly 'horizontal' orientation, which makes a pure

Table 23   Horizontal vs. non-horizontal grating

Method	Year	Duration	Size	Position	Contrast (log ft lamberts)	Results orientation difference
Front projected	1983	150 msec	10° diameter 0.9 cycles/ degree	45° on 45°	Light bars = 0.9	45° = 95% (n = 20)
					Dark bars = 0.68	20° = 85% (n = 20)
					Ground = 0.60	15° = 82.5% (n = 40)
					3 non-test quadrants = 0.95	10° = 75% (n = 20)
						5° = 62.5% (n = 20)

From Weiskrantz and Warrington (in press), by permission.

Table 24   **X** vs. **O**

Method	Year	Duration	Size	Position	Contrast (log ft lamberts)	Results
Back projected	1974/5	2 sec	6.5° × 5.5°	20° on 0°	B on W 1.1/2.0	92.5% (n = 40)
Front projected	1976	125 msec	19° × 12°	25° on 35°	W on B not measured	90% (n = 30)
Front projected	1982	150 msec	9° × 7°	35° on 45°	W on B 0.8/0.0	85% (n = 40)
Front projected	1983	150 msec	10° × 8°	45° on 45°	W on B 0.9/0.6 3 non-test quadrants = 0.95	85% (n = 48) 80% (n = 40)

From Weiskrantz and Warrington (in press), by permission.

test of the hypothesis at the extremes virtually impossible with such a set of stimuli. The matter will be discussed further in Part III and is the subject of a separate paper (Weiskrantz and Warrington, in press), but the present results strongly support the hypothesis that such simple 'form' discrimination as had been previously demonstrated were not based on 'form' as such but on 'orientation'. This position also gains support from the results of 'straight vs. curved triangle' and the 'triangle vs. **X**' tasks, both of which minimize orientation differences between the choice stimuli. He did not score above chance on either of these. For those discriminations that contained a moderate level of orientation cues, his performance itself was only moderate; e.g., the **T** vs. **4** discrimination was approximately at threshold level (75 per cent). In contrast, in the same situations in which these tests were carried out, he

Table 25

Method	Year	Duration	Size	Position	Contrast (log ft lamberts)	Results
			T vs. 4			
Back projected	1975	2 sec	6.2° × 5°	20° on 0°	B on W 1.0/2.0	75% (n = 20)
			X vs. Triangle			
Back projected	1974	2 sec	7.7° × 7.7°	18.7 on 0°	B on W 1.0/2.0	48% (n = 60)
			Straight vs. curved triangle			
Printed cards	1975	2 sec	17° × 17° × 17°	30°, 45°, 60° on 0°	B on W 0.0/0.6	58% (n = 120)
Front projected	1982	150 msec	12° × 12° × 12°	45° on 45°	W on B 0.8/ − 1.1	50% (n = 30)

From Weiskrantz and Warrington (in press), by permission.

Table 26   Square vs. rectangles and diamond

Method	Year	Duration	Size	Position	Contrast (log ft lamberts)	Results
Front projected	1983	150 msec	Square and diamond 7.3° × 7.3° / Rectangle 4.4° × 12.2°	45° on 45°	W on B 0.9/0.6	Square vs. diamond = 87.5% n = 40 / Square vs. rectangle = 60% n = 40
Front projected	1983	150 msec	Square and diamond 7.3° × 7.3° / Rectangle 4.4° × 12.2° / Rectangle 5.1° × 10.4°	45° on 45°	W on B 0.9/0.6	Square vs. diamond = 95% n = 40 / Square vs. rectangle = 85° n = 20 / Square vs. rectangle = 70% n = 40

From Weiskrantz and Warrington (in press), by permission.

could discriminate 'form' stimuli differing in orientation (e.g., he could do **X** vs. **O** almost perfectly even though they were smaller than those 'forms' lacking good orientation cues, on which he failed). 'Pure' orientation discrimination, in the absence of acknowledged awareness (Table 23; cf. also Chapter 7), could also be demonstrated.

9 Detection with slow rate of onset

As has been noted, there were conditions under which D.B. spoke of a feeling of 'movement', 'something coming in from screen', when a stimulus was turned on, at least in certain locations in the visual field. It occurred to us, therefore, to see whether this type of experience would be reported when the stimulus was turned on gradually rather than abruptly, in order to reduce the strength of activity in the 'transient' visual pathways — especially as we have seen patients in whom detection of a stimulus does, indeed, depend upon its onset being very sharp (Weiskrantz 1980). We first tested this very informally with D.B. by mounting an adjustable diaphragm in the path of the light source in the Aimark perimeter. When we turned up the intensity from zero slowly (by hand) and gradually, taking about 3–4 seconds to do so, to our surprise (and his) D.B. jerked backwards, his chin coming off the chin-rest, and exclaimed, 'there was something coming towards me!'

We followed this up, again informally, by mounting a graduated neutral density film on a wheel around the light source aperture in the perimeter, and seeing whether he reported a different impression depending upon whether the intensity was made gradually to increase or decrease. The target (maximum size of the Aimark, 1° 40′) was set at the same intermediate intensity at the beginning of each trial, and randomly either increased or decreased in intensity. The change in intensity was controlled by hand, and the time course was again approximately four seconds. Runs of 30 trials were given, at 75°, 50°, and 25° eccentricity on the horizontal meridian. He was asked whether he had 'a feeling of movement' and if so, whether it was towards or away from him. If uncertain he was required to guess. The result was that at 75° eccentricity he said he had a definite feeling of movement and on all 15 occasions when the light was dimmed he responded 'going away', and on 12 out of the other 15, when it was being made brighter, he said, 'coming towards'. But at the other two eccentricities, 50° and 25°, he said 'just guessing. No feeling of any movement. I was not aware of any light there are all'. At 50° he nevertheless responded even more consistently than he had at the 75° eccentricity, where he had reported an experience: he only once said that a target increasing in intensity was an 'away' trial; in all other cases he responded 'towards' for an increase, and 'away' for a decrease, although he said he was doing it by 'guessing'. That is, if one scores as correct an 'away' response to decrease, and a 'towards' response to increase, he performed at 27/30 and 29/30 at the two positions, respectively.

At the narrowest eccentricity, where he also had no experience, he performed at 20/30, but showed gradual improvement in the run — all but one of the 'errors' were made in the first 15 trials.

These results, although very suggestive, obviously required a firmer control of the temporal and intensity features of the stimulus than was possible in the informal tests. The following report is of experiments in which those requirements were met and applied in tests in April 1982.

An apparatus was constructed in which two polaroid filters were mounted, allowing light to pass through them from the projecting tachistoscope. One of the filters could be rotated mechanically by a motor, the speed of which was closely controlled by a feedback circuit with an input from a photo-cell which monitored the light passing through the filters. The rate of rotation could be varied such that the rise time (or fall) of the light transmitted through the filters could be controlled from 1 msec through several minutes (we are much indebted to Mr. B. Baker of the Oxford Department of Experimental Psychology for the design and construction of the apparatus). The starting and finishing positions of the rotating filter could also be specified in advance, these also controlled by circuitry fed by the photo-cell monitor, by presetting a counter with a range from 0 to 100. The rate of change of the filter was linear with respect to the counter setting. The light level of the target formed by the projector beam passing through the apparatus was measured with the S.E.I. photometer, and is shown in Fig. 27. The curves are shown plotted on a log ft lambert scale and also on a cube root scale, as this is claimed to be a good estimate of the magnitude estimation of brightness as a function of physical intensity (Stevens 1961). The photometer was not sensitive enough to measure the values very near the low end of the curve, but the actual impression of changing brightness was continuous over the whole range, even at the lower region, and in fact phenomenally it appeared to be approximately linear, although formal magnitude estimation was not actually carried out.

The inset panels in the figure show the six conditions that were tested. The rise time was set to be 1 msec (A, D in Fig. 27), 2000 msec (B, E), or 10 000 msec (C, F), and the maximum light level to be either 1000 (A, B, C) or 200 (D, E, F) on the scale (-0.17 log ft lamberts or -1.21 log ft lamberts). The target was a circular disc, 10° diameter, placed with its centre 25° eccentric on the 45° lower left meridian. The room was that of the 'standard situation', except that because of the lower maximum intensity of the target imposed by the polaroid filters (the filters reduced the maximum level of the projected target by just over 2 log units), the background level was also reduced by having only one background projector on, and it illuminated the upper left quadrant, producing a level of -1.65 log ft lamberts there. The level of the lower left test quadrant was the same as the minimum level of target intensity, approximately -1.8 log ft lamberts.

D.B. was given the same instructions as for any presence/absence procedure, except that he was told that the signal would not be instantaneous

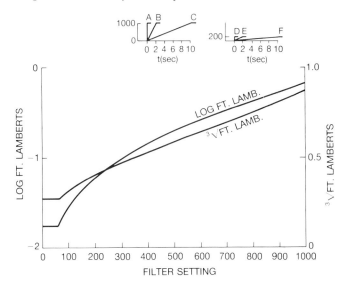

Fig. 27. Calibration curve for light levels against filter setting in gradual onset experiment, in log ft lamberts and also as cube root function to approximate apparent brightness (Stevens 1961). Filter changed linearly with time to one of two different maximum brightness levels, as shown in insets at top. D.B.'s scores were as follows: A = 95%; B = 90%; C = 85%; D = 87.5%: E = 87.5%; F = 85%. (See text for further details)

in all conditions. He was to respond 'yes' if the target was present or 'no' if not, but not to make his response until signalled to do so by the experimenter. (The sequence was 'ready' just before the trial, 'now' at the beginning, and 'OK' when required to respond. The target, if there was one, was kept on until he gave his response to the 'OK' command, and then switched off). On half of the trials, on a quasi-random schedule, the target was not presented (by blocking the light path from the projector with an opaque occluder), although of course all the components of the apparatus were operated in the same way on all trials. In the first three blocks (20 trials each) the target went from the minimum to the maximum level in the first block, in 1 msec (Fig. 27, A), in the second block in 2000 msec (B), and in the third block in 10 000 msec (C). His performance was, respectively, 19/20, 18/20, and 17/20 correct, all errors throughout being failures to detect the target.

Because he may have been limited by a ceiling effect, we then reduced the maximum light level achieved by the target to 200 on the scale, and presented six more blocks, in the order 2000 (E), 10 000 (F), 1 (D), 1 (D), 10 000 (F), and 2000 msec (E). His overall scores were 35/40 for the 1 msec condition, 35/40 for the 2000 msec condition, and 34/40 for the 10 000 condition, all errors again being false negatives. Thus, as in the informal tests, he was able to detect at well above chance levels a target with a slow onset, even when it was for a change in target illumination of only 0.6 log units spread over 10 000 msec, and to do so with only a slight reduction in accuracy compared with an abrupt onset.

Verbal commentaries

When the light level of the target was increased over its maximum range, he said he had 'a feeling of movement a couple of times' during the 1 msec condition (A). In the 2000 msec condition (B), he said that there was sometimes a small movement, but he thought he performed at a 'little more than 50:50'. In the slowest condition (C), he reported only that 'when I said 'yes' I wanted to say "yes" before you asked me (to respond)'.

When the maximum light level was reduced to a scale value of 200 (-1.21 log ft lamberts) he said for the 1 msec condition (D), 'I got a movement quite often, and said "yes" when I did. I was quite confident'. His response for the 2000 msec condition (E) was ambiguous. He said 'I knew I was right *after* I spoke'. 'When I said "yes" I knew a couple of seconds after that I got it right'. (This presumably referred to the feed-back he had from the abrupt termination of a target after he had made his response.) Thus, both an abrupt onset or offset produced a report of an experience, although the slower onset as such did not. Finally, in the slowest condition (F), he said for the first block, 'I was just above chance'. For the second block, he said, 'I didn't do very well. Just guess work, 50:50. No movement at all'. Thus, as in informal testing, whether or not he performed well did not depend on nor did it correlate with his reported experience.

Comment

An ability to respond reliably to a stimulus that takes 10 seconds to reach its full value of 0.6 log units above the initial value (= background level), gradually and smoothly, is a demanding test of his capacity to respond to a 'non-transient' event. Of course, one cannot rule out transients introduced by eye movement tremor during fixation, but at least it is clear that D.B.'s capacity is quite different from those described by Riddoch (1917), for example, for whom it was said stimuli could not be detected unless there was vigorous and definite movement of the target. D.B. is clearly able to detect stationary stimuli even when they are introduced very gradually. Of course, as he does not necessarily acknowledge any awareness of such stimuli, as we have seen, it is quite possible that patients described by Riddoch would also be able to carry out the same task as D.B. if required to make forced-choice responses, even though they, too, might not 'see' them. But that is another issue. What is clear here is that first-order transients are not necessary for D.B.'s capacity to detect, as such, although they *may* be a necessary condition for an experience of change.

10 The natural blind-spot (optic disc) within the scotoma

The optic disc provides a ready-made control for determining the discriminable limits of intra-ocular diffusion. As the size of this natural and absolutely blind area is fixed and known ($5° \times 7°$), a target light that cannot be detected by the subject when it is positioned on the optic disc cannot cause detectable diffusion beyond a maximum angle determined by the distance between the edge of the target and the nearest region of sensitive retina. (This value is probably an overestimate of intra-ocular diffusion, because the disc itself is more highly reflective than the rest of the retina, and hence is a more effective diffuser of light.)

The rationale of the experiment was to compare detection of a small target when it fell on the objectively blind disc with detection in a number of neighbouring locations within the scotoma. The procedure was carried out in April 1982, and results were as follows (Weiskrantz and Warrington, in press; a brief reference also appears in Weiskrantz 1983).

We first adjusted the lighting and target conditions so that a target on the optic disc disappeared completely and without any 'halo'. Under the same conditions we then located the optic disc in D.B.'s *intact* right half-field, with the left eye masked; the target was small (33′) with a light value of 1.15 log ft lamberts, 2 seconds duration. The luminance of the background on the Aimark perimeter was not measured, but was estimated to be -1.0 log ft lamberts. With forced-choice guessing, D.B. performed at chance over 40 trials, with the target at an eccentricity of 16° on a meridian just below (3°–4°) the horizontal meridian. The right eye was then masked, and a mirror symmetrical position in the left field was tested with the same target, as well as two other positions. The target was presented among the three positions in an order fixed by a Latin square, as follows: 25°, disc, 10°, disc, 10°, 25°, 10°, 25°, and disc. In each location, 10 trials were given before proceeding to the next location, giving a total of 30 trials per location. The results were as follows: on the disc: 43 per cent (chance). At 10°: 90 per cent. At 25°: 97 per cent.

Next, using the same target, we probed three more locations in the scotoma along another meridian, 60° below horizontal. Thirty trials at eccentricities of 45°, 30°, and 15° were tested, in that order. The results were: At 45°: 77 per cent. At 30°: 90 per cent. At 15°: 93 per cent. The results for his performance at all locations tested is shown in Figure 28.

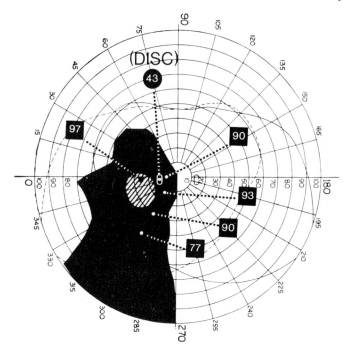

Fig. 28. Results of optic disc experiment. Numbers in insets show per cent correct in 30 trials for forced-choice detection (chance = 50%) at different locations, including the optic disc, for a 0.5° target. The scotoma was plotted in the same apparatus, but a high contrast and large 1° 40′ target so that any bias would be in the direction of underestimating the size of the field defect. The hatching indicates estimates area within which D.B. had a 'feeling' of stimulus presentation. See text for further details. (Redrawn from Weiskrantz 1983, by permission)

Thus, D.B. was able to detect a target in the scotoma but not in the 'blind-spot' within the scotoma. As the target's diffusion must be less than 2¼°, his success at detection in the scotoma is not adequately accounted for by diffusion of light from within the scotoma to a sensitive region of retina outside the scotoma, as has been suggested by Campion *et al.* (1983).

Verbal commentaries

He was questioned carefully after each block of ten trials. At all locations, except one, he consistently and insistently said that he was 'just guessing'. For example, at the 15° eccentricity, on the 60° lower left meridian, he said, 'it's a dead area. No sensation. Just guessing'. Q: 'Like tossing a coin?' A: 'Yes'. (He performed at 28/30 = 93 per cent). The one exceptional location was at the 25° eccentricity in the 4° to 5° off-horizontal meridian. After each of the 3 blocks of trials, his comment was similar: 'I feel something coming in', and he expressed confidence in his judgements. The region within which he felt some sort of movement was not measured directly for this size and contrast of target, but by extrapolation was roughly estimated to occupy the hatched area in Fig. 28. These reports are similar to those experiences, when they occurred, that he reported for Aimark targets in certain locations in the field using other procedures, e.g., presence/absence, and reaching.

Comment

This test is a very stringent one for demonstrating the insufficiency of stray light as an explanation of D.B.'s ability to detect stimuli in his scotoma. The maximum detectable spread of light is $2\frac{1}{4}°$, as judged by the chance performance for the target on the disc. All of the non-disc positions in the scotoma yielded above chance performance, and all were greater than this distance from the nearest region of intact field. As regards his reported experience of 'feeling' in one region of the scotoma, the general question of the conditions and the area over which such experiences may emerge will be dealt with more fully in Part III. Here it is worth noting, again, that his ability to detect, as such, does not depend upon there being a reported experience. Nor, it is important to note, did he distinguish at all between his lack of experience when the target fell on the genuine blind-spot, and when it fell on the four positions that were in the 'dead' field: in all these cases he felt or saw nothing, and said he was just guessing; during the Latin square design the blocks of disc and non-disc trials were intermixed. The importance of this outcome lies in the comparison that can be made directly between the positive residual capacity of the scotoma and that of a region that can objectively be defined as 'blind'. Subjectively there was no reported difference between the objectively blind region and the neighbouring 'dead' area of the scotoma. It was only in terms of objective discriminative capacity that the scotoma and the optic disc were different.

11   Left versus right eye

On a number of occasions when the two eyes were compared it was seen that the left eye seemed better than the right. This was true with discrimination of orientation, and also with 'presence/absence'. The question also arose in discussion of double dissociation of form and detection, when it was found that the impaired field was paradoxically better than the good field in a detection task at an extreme eccentricity (80°). Because stimuli at this eccentricity fall within the monocular crescent, it is possible that this surprising result of 'super-normal' performance in the impaired field might actually reflect a sub-normal performance of the unimpaired field because of its constricted pupil that resulted from the right cervical sympathectomy. In August 1983 we explored this possibility.

Method

One way to investigate the matter is to test sensitivity with viewing through an artificial pupil. This was done by securely taping a thin copper foil, in which a small circular aperture was cut, to D.B.'s eyebrow and cheek. The hole was fixed so that it allowed a viewing angle of 30° between the fixation point at one edge and the stimulus, at the opposite edge. Under the conditions of ambient illumination in the 'standard situation', the pupil of D.B.'s right eye was approximately 4.0 mm. The pupil of the left eye was noticeably larger, but not measured. A series of aperture sizes were prepared; a 4.0 mm aperture in the foil was found to be the smallest that would allow a viewing angle of 30° between the fixation and the stimulus at the standard viewing distance of 1 metre. The threshold for detection of the 10° diameter disc of the 'standard situation' was first measured for each eye with the artificial pupil, and then without the artificial pupil, using the staircase method.

Results

Viewed through the artificial pupil the left eye had a threshold of 2.35 log units of attention, and the right eye a threshold of 2.25 log units. There was much overlap between the values for the two eyes, and in fact the first value at which each eye reached its first threshold value was the same: 2.3 log units. Without the artificial pupil, the left eye's threshold was 2.80, the right's was 2.45. Here there was no overlap. The left eye went below threshold at 2.7, 2.9, 2.8, and 2.9 log units, the right at 2.5, 2.5, 2.5, and 2.5 log units.

And so the left eye's advantage, while it had a marginal but insignificant advantage with the artificial pupil, was distinctly greater without the artificial pupil. While more exacting tests of the question would be useful, the results do support the interpretation that D.B.'s superior performance with his left eye and in his far peripheral left field with binocular vision derived from the constricted pupil of the right eye.

12 Detection of direction of contrast

Because D.B., when he acknowledges having some sort of impression or feeling when a stimulus is abruptly presented, fails to ascribe any sense of 'brightness' to the experience—in fact, on one occasion he said, 'it is as though I imagine that I am moving my finger in front of my eyes in the dark'—it seemed possible that he would be unable to respond to the contrast of a stimulus on the ground. That is, he might treat a black spot on a grey ground as equivalent to a white spot on the same ground. We put this to the test in February 1975. Two grey cards were prepared, $24° \times 17°$ in size, with a small black or white square, $3.6° \times 3.6°$, positioned in the centre. The cards were clipped to the Aimark perimeter at an eccentricity of 45° on the horizontal meridian. They were covered by a masking card, removed for a period of two seconds during each trial. The overhead fluorescent lamps were on, giving a light level on the card of 0.70 log ft lamberts. The level of the black square was 0 log ft lamberts, and of the white square, 1.1 log ft lamberts.

It was necessary to establish, first of all, that D.B. could detect the presence of a spot as such. He was asked to judge 'spot' or 'no spot', the spot consisting of the black spot described above. He scored 18/20 correct. He was then given two blocks of 20 trials in which he was presented with either the white or the black spot, and asked to judge which it was. He scored 17/20 and 18/20 correct. Therefore, at least under these conditions, he has no difficulty in discriminating direction of contrast.

Verbal commentary

He described his judgement as being based not on the brightness of any impression, but on its nearness to him. 'When I said "white" it seemed like something close. When I said "black" it seemed like something further away'. This type of comment is consistent with his remarks during presence/absence and other judgements, where the felt 'closeness' of an object 'coming out of the screen' seems to vary with the amount by which it is brighter than the background.

13 'Waves'

In testing in 1982 (cf., for example, the Chapter 10 tests on the optic disc within the scotoma), but especially in 1983, D.B. reported an impression of 'waves' in parts of his field defect, especially in a region between the fovea and about 30° eccentric in the lower quadrant. The region had been plotted in Fig. 27 in Chapter 10. In 1983 we recorded our impression that his 'live' field was livelier and slightly larger than before. The experience is of a kind unlike anything in normal visual experience, and for which precise words seem to be lacking. The 'waves' can have some sort of form. They can be straight or curved, or can even have a 'squareness'. They can also be 'quick', which is how he described one of the Aimark targets in a reaching experiment. 'A quick movement; not a light'. The square was described as producing 'a sharp movement'. He also described the square on another occasion as producing 'a corner-shaped wave'. The waves could also be thinner or thicker, e.g., in the uncurved triangle vs. curved triangle discrimination, he said, 'There is a movement. I said "straight" when the waves are thinner, and "curved" when they are thicker and quicker'. But D.B. insisted that he was not *seeing*. Interestingly, he mentioned in 1983 that he experiences these waves in everyday life. If, for example, there is a moving cat in his field defect, this sets up waves of the same sort that he experiences when having a migraine attack. He said that he cannot be sure, in such a situation, whether or not he is having a migraine attack until the cat emerges into his good visual field! The sensitivity would also seem to be quite high, and can be induced by his own movement. For example, he said that when he is walking at dusk, he is unable to see on his right side because of the darkness, but his left side of the field is intrusive because it contains waves.

It is not surprising that the properties of such an experience, when present, could provide the basis for a discrimination if they seem to flip from one state to another during a two-choice run in a successive discrimination. Equally, if they are unstable, they might be distracting. Or, if they have been used as the basis of a choice and then no longer occur, discrimination might suffer until D.B. is able to switch to a 'non-wave' mode. Or, a stimulus might occur partially in the 'live' field and partially outside it; the 'waves' set up by a corner of either a square or a rectangle might be used for attempting a discrimination, which could, of course, be inadequate. We saw examples of all of these phenomena, as judged by the comments that D.B. made after runs of trials. For example, in a series of runs in 1983 with the diamond vs.

square discrimination, he reported differential types of 'moving waves' with the two stimuli when they fell at an eccentricity of 28°, and then at 35°. When the stimuli were moved to a more extreme eccentricity, 40°, the waves disappeared. His performance immediately fell to chance. But, in fact, as will be seen, if he is not actually attending to or searching for waves, the same discrimination can readily be made at a high level in the 'dead' field.

Similarly, the waves can be misleading. In 1983, in fact, we first became aware of the increasing liveliness of parts of his field when we tested his reaching performance in the Aimark perimeter. His performance was more erratic than it had been previously, and he mentioned the 'little dart-like movements' which seemed to be localized on a plane *other* than the perimeter arc. Also, in one of the straight vs. curved triangle runs in 1983, he pointed to an impression of waves at the apex of the stimuli, which was common to both stimuli.

In August 1983 we took special pains to see whether discrimination could still be displayed even when the 'waves' were abolished. This was done by directing stimuli to the 'dead' part of the field and, by using low contrast stimuli, to restrict their influence spatially. The particular findings are also described in the relevant sections (cf. Tables 23, 24, 25, 26), but are usefully put into a single perspective here.

The principal manoeuvres were to increase the ambient level of illumination on the test quadrant by using bright overhead fluorescent lamps in the standard testing room (see Chapter 17), which raised the level by 1.72 log units to 0.60 log ft lamberts, and also to place the stimuli eccentrically. The flooding projectors were still directed to the other three quadrants, which had an ambient level of 0.95 log ft lamberts. The centres of the stimuli were directed to a location 45° eccentric on the lower 45° meridian, and their light level measured 0.90 log ft lamberts. Under these conditions, D.B. consistently (and insistently) reported no experience of any kind: 'nothing there. All guess-work' or similar comments after every single run. He was able, nevertheless, to score 95 per cent correct on the square vs. diamond discrimination. In contrast, it was in that same condition that his performance was relatively degraded when orientation was removed as a cue from a 'form' discrimination, i.e., square vs. rectangle.

Orientation discrimination was also measured under the same 'dead' conditions. The results were especially surprising, because in the previous year for the same position in the field but under conditions of high contrast and low background levels, D.B. was unable to succeed in doing even a 90° discrimination. In the present low contrast condition, the ambient light levels were as indicated just above. The level of the white bar in the grating was 0.90 log ft lamberts, and of the dark bar 0.68 log ft lamberts. (Note that the white bar is approximately the same level as the three surrounding quadrants.) As in the 'standard situation' a square wave grating was used, occupying a circular field of 10° diameter, with a spatial frequency of 0.9 cycles/degree.

D.B. was given runs of horizontal vs. 15°, 15°, 10°, 5°, 20°, and 45°, in that order, and performed well for all differences of greater than 10°. At that point, he scored 75 per cent (15/20), which is threshold value, and at 5°, he fell to 13/20. His threshold value of 10° is better than any other score he has achieved for an orientation discrimination with gratings in his impaired field, and compares well with his threshold at that eccentricity in his good half-field.

Although, as we have seen, performance in the absence of any subjective experience can be superior to that resulting from stimuli placed in a 'live' part of the field, when such 'waves' are present they can scarcely be ignored. Whether they help or not depends, as we have indicated, on their precise correspondence to the demands of the discrimination. But the present results not only demonstrate, once again, that acknowledged experience was not a prerequisite for impressive discriminative performance by D.B., but also, as the conditions employed high ambient levels of illumination and low contrast stimuli, they serve to reinforce those control procedures that rule out an explanation in terms of diffusion of light within the eye or stray light.

It is a moot point whether the picture would not have been fuller and more revealing had we used high ambient levels for a greater range of tests, especially in the period prior to the contraction of the field defect in 1976. Because one assumed (correctly) that D.B.'s detection threshold was somewhat elevated, one was always swayed by the natural impulse to try to make the stimuli as distinctive and salient as possible, with high contrast, short of allowing artefacts to intrude from diffusion of light. And the verbal reports of several sections reveal how curious non-visual experiences might result, which could also have biased D.B. himself towards seeking such a basis for his discriminations and against settling for a non-experiential mode. We had been struck early on in our tests with D.B. that he was able to settle down into such a mode with some ease. After one long session, when we feared he might have become as fatigued as the experimenters had become in the arduous task of presenting long runs of stimuli in random sequence, he explained that he was not at all tired. 'I am not doing anything', he said! In contrast, when he was carrying out psychophysical judgements in his good field, he showed the fatigue that is customary in such a procedure. It might have been salutary to have always arranged conditions to be quite 'dead'.

The evidence is obviously not sufficient to support speculation as to whether the 'live' part of the field reflects partially functioning areas of striate cortex, or possibly an irritative phenomenon or, what may also be a related phenomenon, denervation super-sensitivity of partially disconnected striate cortex. Equally, the dead part of the field may reflect a total dysfunction of striate cortex or, alternatively, remnants of striate cortex at an even lower level of dysfunction than the 'live' levels. Given the animal and other evidence, we favour a view that relies on midbrain pathways, but the issue will be discussed at greater length in Part III.

14 Matching between impaired and intact fields

If, as the results of the double dissociation between form and detection suggest, the impaired field is qualitatively different from the normal field, the interesting question arises whether communication between the two fields is possible and, if so, is efficient. The way we have approached this question is to present stimuli to the two fields simultaneously and ask D.B. to make a 'same-different' judgement. Two groups of such tests have been carried out, in September 1975, and in April 1982.

On the first occasion, the stimuli used were curved and straight triangles, the same photographic prints which have been described in Chapter 8 (intermediate size, each side of straight triangle between 16° and 28°). The stimuli were mounted on the Aimark perimeter at an eccentricity of 45° on the horizontal meridian of each field. The light level of the white background of the cards was 0.60 log ft lamberts. The stimuli were covered with masking cards, which were removed for two seconds for presentation in each trial. On every trial stimuli were presented in both fields; on half of the occasions the two fields contained the same stimuli, and on the other half, different ones, and D.B. had to respond simply 'same' or 'different'. Half of the stimulus population were straight, the other half curved triangles (C-7).

On two blocks of 24 trials each, D.B. scored 17/24 and 12/24 correct, or 60 per cent correct. He was then given a further 24 trials of a presumably simpler task, namely straight triangles vs. a blank card, again at 45° eccentricity. He scored 17/24 correct = 71 per cent. But this experiment is ambiguous because it is not clear that he would have been able to discriminate straight vs. curved triangles when presented to the left field alone; the results at this eccentricity have been marginal (see Chapter 8).

But his *verbal commentaries* on this task were surprisingly discrepant with his actual performance. On the two runs of curved vs. straight triangles, he said of the first run, 'I think I got 90 per cent correct. They balance or do not match up. I just *know*'. After the second run, when he performed exactly at chance, he said 'I reckon I got about 99 out of 100'. After the easier triangle vs. blank matching task, he said, 'I am pretty confident. Probably got all right except one. I should have changed my mind on one'.

The second set of tests (in April 1982) used **X**s and **O**s flashed by the tachistoscopic projector for a duration of 150 msec. They were first presented at 25° eccentricity, on the lower 45° meridian in each half-field. The size of the **X** was 5.9° high × 4.7° wide. The **O** was 6.5° high × 5.9° wide. The contrast was light on dark. The lighting conditions were as for the 'standard situation', except that, of course, the projectors for both the lower left *and* right quadrants were equated during the two-field experiments. During presentations to the left field alone, the lower right field was again masked by the two background projectors as usual. The ambient levels were − 1.05 log ft lamberts on the test quadrants, and 0.4 log ft lamberts on the upper two quadrants. The level of the light portion of the stimuli was 0.8 log ft lamberts, with a background of 0 log ft lamberts during the stimulus presentation.

D.B. was first given a block of 10 trials of **X** vs. **O** in the left field alone to establish whether he was at least capable of performing the discrimination there. He was — he scored 100 per cent correct. He was then given two runs of 20 trials on the matching task. Stimuli were always presented in both fields, half of them same, half of them different. Half were **X** and half **O**. He scored 17/20 and 17/20 = 85 per cent.

The next question was whether he would be able to perform so well at a wider eccentricity, 35°, where the form discrimination results suggested he would be able to discriminate **X** vs. **O** but without any accompanying experience when they were flashed. We started by trying the same absolute size of stimuli as had been used in the previous two runs (but because of their greater eccentricity on the tangent screen, their angular size was slightly smaller, $\mathbf{X} = 4.9° \times 3.9°$; $\mathbf{O} = 5.4° \times 4.8°$). We first presented them to the left field alone to establish whether they were discriminable there. They were not: he performed only 4/10. Therefore, the stimuli were increased in size to $\mathbf{X} = 9.5° \times 7.3°$; $\mathbf{O} = 9.3° \times 8.3°$. Given four blocks of 10 trials in the left field alone, he scored 9/10, 9/10, 8/10, and 8/10 = 85 per cent overall. And so the stimuli were now presented to the two fields simultaneously for the matching task proper. He was given two blocks of 20 trials. On the first he achieved 17/20, but on the second only 11/20. At this stage we thought he was showing definite signs of fatigue, and so we once again tested his left field alone. He scored only 9/20 (in contrast to the 85 per cent earlier in the session) and we therefore discontinued the tests, to resume them on the following day.

In those follow-up tests, we continued to monitor the performance of the left field alone during the course of the two-field matching experiments. Using the same larger size stimuli as had just been used previously, at the same eccentricity (35°), we presented blocks of 12 trials in the following order: L + R, L only, L only, L + R, L only, L + R, L + R, L only. His performance was satisfactorily maintained throughout. His scores were as follows: L + R, 9/12, 9/12, 9/12, and 9/12 = 75 per cent overall. L only: 8/12, 10/12, 11/12, and 12/12 = 85.4 per cent. Thus, he showed unmistakable evidence of being able to do the matching task, if only at moderate levels of performance. His ability to do the discrimination within the left field alone was better than across fields, although only by virtue of his gradual improvement of the within-field task as testing proceeded. (In any case, the two-field task is presumably a more difficult one than the one-field task.) A question arises, of course, as to how he succeeded. It is possible that he carried out the task sequentially. As he could discriminate the stimuli in each field independently, he could have provided himself with a verbal label for each. The question will be considered later.

Verbal commentaries for Xs and Os

The stimuli when presented to the left field alone at 25° eccentricity (in the preliminary run in which he scored 10/10 at that position) did produce reported experiences: 'There were two different shapes—one is thick and round, the other not so thick, not so round. There is a wave—I'm not *seeing*. There is something coming in'. But during the two-field matching runs at this eccentricity, when he performed at 85 per cent correct, he said that he was 'not aware of anything on the left, but I see it on the right'. In the first run, he thought he had performed at 'a little bit above chance', but in the second run he was 'confident—got 99 per cent correct', although he continued to report that he 'noticed nothing on the left'.

We switched to the wider eccentricity, as has been intimated, to see whether performance could be maintained when there was no longer any experience of the stimuli presented to the left field alone. In this we succeeded. During the four runs with the stimuli in the left field alone, when he performed at 85 per cent, he said throughout: 'just guessing—50:50. I did not even know the light was on'. And later, 'same as before—just guessing'. During the two-field matching tests that followed, as well as during the blocks when the stimuli were presented to the left field alone, his response continued the same: 'saw nothing on the left—pure guess-work. 50:50'. 'Just guessing. No sense of anything coming in'. On the final run of trials with the stimuli presented only to the left field, when he scored *100 per cent*, he said 'just a terrible score—it's got to be 50:50 or worse'. Thus, as with other stimuli, discrimination in the 'blind' field can be carried out at a high level in the absence of acknowledged awareness. Similarly, under all conditions in which he succeeded in this **X** vs. **O** two-field matching task, he reported no experience, although he maintained a moderate and stable level of performance at 75 per cent. There is no ready explanation for the contrast between the situation with **X** vs. **O** two-field experiments, where he did reasonably well but reported no awareness of anything (in the left field) and had no confidence, and the earlier tests with curved vs. straight triangles— when he performed poorly but was extremely confident that he was succeeding. But the contrast provides a further example of a dissociation between performance and subjective report.

15 Matching within the impaired field

As we have seen, matching between stimuli in the impaired and the mirror-symmetrical normal field is possible for D.B., at least for **X** vs. **O**, at a moderate level of success. But, as mentioned, it is possible that the performance was carried out successively. That is, it is already clear that he can make a successive discrimination between these two stimuli when they are projected singly in the impaired field. To store what was presented in the good field for a short interval while making a decision about the impaired field would not be a demanding task, and would enable a match to be made efficiently. The matter could, perhaps, be pursued by careful analysis of reaction times in the single vs. double field presentations.

A further and more interesting question arises regarding the question of matching of pairs of stimuli that fall entirely within the impaired field. This was investigated in August 1983.

Method

D.B. sat 1 metre from the screen used in the 'standard condition'. The stimuli were arranged to fall to either side of the 45° meridian in the lower left quadrant, such that the nearest point of the **X** or the **O** to the 45° meridian was approximately 5°. The centres were at an eccentricity of 33° from the fixation point. The stimuli were projected for a duration of 150 msec. and consisted of a bright figure on a darker ground. They were projected in an upright orientation, and their sizes were 22×19 cm for the **O**, approximately $10° \times 8°$, and 20×15 cm for the **X**, approximately $9° \times 7°$. The overhead lights were on, and in addition there were projectors illuminating the three other quadrants, as in the arrangement for the 'standard situation'. Each of these three quadrants had a light reading of 0.95 log ft lamberts, while the lower left test quadrant had a background level of 0.60 log ft lamberts. The light level of the stimuli figures was 0.90 log ft lamberts. The overhead lights plus quadrant projectors were intended to reduce the intrusive effects of the 'waves' of which D.B. complained at this stage of testing.

Results

It was first necessary to see whether he could discriminate **X** from **O** presented singly. He was given 20 trials for the position just above the 45° meridian and another 20 trials for the position just below it. He scored 19/20 and 20/20 correct respectively. He was then given stimuli in both positions simultaneously, and was asked to judge 'same' or 'different'. (The sequence of pairs were constructed from pairs of rows of the Gellerman tables). He scored 9/20 and 10/20 correct.

Because, under these conditions at least, D.B. clearly was unable to perform a comparison for stimuli falling within the impaired field, it was important to show that this was not due simply to the task being too difficult *per se*. The same task was carried out in the mirror symmetric position in the good field, and he scored 100 per cent out of 10 trials and he commented that it was 'easy'. The task was also done by one of us (EKW), who made no errors and found it easy to do.

Verbal commentaries

From the stimuli in the impaired field, when presented singly, D.B. reported 'not very much of an impression. I said "O" when I got a slight bending wave—"X" when I got nothing at all'. He said he felt confident. For the paired stimuli in the matching condition, he also reported 'bent waves'. He felt 'fairly confident. I think I did a little better than 50:50'. It was because of D.B.'s comments about the intrusion of 'waves' for certain stimuli in particular parts of the impaired field that we deliberately raised the background luminance and reduced the contrast, as also reported for certain other procedures, because he seemed to perform better when he was completely devoid of experience (e.g., see results of diamonds vs. squares in Chapter 8; also Chapter 7 for August 1983. The matter is discussed in Chapter 13).

Comment

There was a marked difference between the results of the between-field and within-field matching experiments. He could succeed in the former but not in the latter. Admittedly, the two were carried out under somewhat different conditions of luminance, and the tasks also differ in terms of difficulty and other respects. Because of the theoretical implications the matter deserves further work, e.g., varying the spatial separation between the pairs, the formal properties of the stimuli, perhaps attempting a numerosity judgement, but given the utterly simple level of the present within-field task and its undemanding character when done in the normal visual field, as far as they go the results are striking.

16 Double dissociations between form and detection

Given that the existence of many features of residual visual capacity in D.B. was undetected by clinical examination or his own experience, it would hardly be surprising if his residual visual capacity was normal quantitatively. Leaving aside the question of his own awareness of his capacity, most of the objective measures reveal at least some loss compared to visual thresholds in his good right half-field. But the question is whether the residual function is qualitatively similar to normal vision — merely degraded in its capacity — or whether there are differences in *kind*. One's impression, no doubt fostered as well by animal evidence and 'two visual system' theorizing, is that his ability to discriminate or identify forms, especially those that cannot be reduced to another type of discrimination, may be degraded disproportionately in relation to his ability to detect, to locate, or to discriminate orientations. One valuable approach to the question of whether there are qualitative differences is to see whether it is possible to demonstrate double dissociation of function, i.e., whether there are some conditions under which the left field is relatively superior to the right and others under which the opposite is true.

We chose to compare measures of detection and form discrimination in the two half-fields, and we have made quantitative comparisons in two separate experiments. The first was in October 1974. The strategy was to find a location in his good half-field at which detection was *inferior* to that in his impaired field, and then to examine his capacity to perform a shape discrimination at that position. When using a sine-wave grating of fixed spatial frequency and contrast (generated by the Ives diffraction apparatus used for acuity, see above) one would expect the performance to fall below threshold beyond a certain retinal eccentricity from the fovea, and we therefore first identified an eccentricity in the good field where his ability to detect the presence or absence of the grating was inferior to that of his impaired field at a less eccentric location. We used a spatial frequency of 1 cycle per degree, at a distance from the eye of 40.7 cm. The other stimulus from which it was discriminated was the 'uniform' field, actually a grating set at a very high value of spatial frequency, indiscriminable from a uniform field even with normal foveal fixation. The grating was presented in a circular aperture 8.9° in diameter. The photometric reading of the uniform field was 2 log ft lamberts. At an eccentricity (along the horizontal meridian) of 73° from the fixation point to the centre of the grating in his *good* field, using

104 Blindsight: a case study and implications

forced-choice responses between 'lines' and 'no lines', he performed at chance (15/30) and also said that he 'saw no lines'.

Having found a location at which detection was poor, in the next block of trials we gave him a discrimination between a triangle and an **X** at the same location. The Ives apparatus was used to back-illuminate the black figures, shaped from black plastic tape and mounted on glass plates, with the dimensions and the procedure as described above (Chapter 8). The **X** was $7.7° × 7.7°$ and the triangle $7.7°$ along each side, with a thickness of each form of $1.9°$. The background photometric conditions were the same for the Ives grating and the triangle vs. **X**. D.B. had no difficulty in discriminating these two shapes in his good field. In 30 trials, he was perfect for the first 20, but made three errors in the last 10 trials ($27/30 = 90\%$). He said that he 'lost 4 or 5 of the last few trials because my eyes started to water' (the 2 log ft lambert light travel is moderately high).

We then switched to the impaired half-field. It had already been established on the preceding day that he was able to detect a 1 cycle per degree grating in a region of the field somewhat beyond $6°$ eccentricity. But we wished to find a location at which his performance with the grating was as near optimal as practicable, in order to put the question to the strongest challenge. We tested various loci with the 1 cycle per degree setting. At $53°$ eccentricity (from centre of grating to fixation point), he scored 22/30, at $45°$, 15/30, at $32°$, 22/30. At $18.2°$ eccentricity, he performed at 28/30. Then, keeping the apparatus at this position, we gave two blocks of form discrimination trials, and finally another block of trials with the grating. The result was that on the triangle vs. cross discrimination he performed at chance (14/30 and $15/30 = 48\%$). On the two blocks of grating trials, his scores were 28/30 and $26/30 = 90$ per cent. After each of these conditions, he said it was 'all guess-work' — both for gratings and forms (although in the final grating block, after he was asked how he had done, he said, 'I am more confident than last time. Perhaps I scored 20/30'). On the other three blocks, including the first grating block, he expressed no confidence at all, and thought he had performed no better than at '50:50, chance'.

Thus, at a location in his impaired field where he was reliably sensitive for detection of a grating, he was unable to discriminate the forms. At a location in his good field where, because of its wide eccentricity from fixation, he was unable to detect the grating, he is still able to perform the same form discrimination with high efficiency (see Table 27, top).

The second experiment also used a peripheral location in the good field ($80°$ eccentricity along the horizontal meridian) at which to test detection and form, but the same eccentricity was also used in the impaired field. The form discrimination consisted of the straight vs. curved triangles (see Chapter 8) used earlier in the same sessions in September 1975. The detection task was a simple 'presence vs. absence' discrimination, using the smallest and weakest stimulus available with the Aimark perimeter. In a pilot run, we first wished to see whether the form discrimination was possible at such a far peripheral location in the good field. Using the easiest discrimination in the set (C-7 vs. straight triangle) he seemed to be capable of the task at a moderate level of success, 21/30. We therefore embarked on the formal run of tests. In the good field we first tested form, and then detection. We then switched to the impaired field and tested detection, then form. Finally, we returned to the good field and once again tested form. Various control procedures were also inserted at certain stages, as will be described.

The light level was relatively low throughout the tests, but the contrast for the detection test was also low. The Aimark arc gave a reading of -1.8 log ft lamberts. The black outline triangles were on white photographic paper, clipped to the Aimark arc, and with a reading of -1.0 log ft lamberts. The size of the triangles was the same as the intermediate size used before, e.g., each side $>16° <28°$. The size of the spot used for detection testing was the smallest and dimmest available in the perimeter, namely 10' in diameter, and with a light value of -0.60 log ft lamberts. The stimulus duration throughout was two seconds.

In the first formal block of the test for form discrimination in the good field at 80° eccentricity, D.B. scored 86.7 per cent (26/30). We then tested his presence vs. absence discrimination in the same field. As he said he did not see the light, we instructed him to guess. In two successive blocks, he scored 68.3 per cent (21/30 and 20/30). We then inserted a control procedure to check for an artefact that might have been caused by the sound of the 'silent' Aimark switch. The light was turned off throughout one whole block, but the switch operated normally as though one were presenting light trials and not 'blanks'. He scored 19/30. We then gave another run in which, again, all trials were 'blanks' but the silent switch was never used. He scored 14/30. We then returned to using the switch, but again with all trials consisting of 'blanks', and he scored 21/30. Finally, we gave one more experimental set of trials, 50 per cent light–no light, using the switch, and he scored 23/30. The outcome of these procedures was, therefore, that he scored 64/90 (71%) when lights were actually presented. The control procedure, however, when lights were never presented, but the same switching was used, yielded a score 40/60 (67%). As the score dropped to a strictly chance level, 14/30, when the switch was not used, it seems reasonable to conclude that the switch probably did, in fact, introduce an artefact; although not a strong signal, it was capable of introducing a false increment of about 20 per cent above the chance level. Compared to that control level, it also seems reasonable to conclude that D.B. was, in fact, correct in saying that he could not detect the light — his score was only four per cent above the level that emerged from the control test. (It was as a result of this control procedure that we abandoned the use of the Aimark switching arrangement in subsequent detection tests (see Chapter 4).

When we turned to the same eccentricity in the impaired field, however, the results for detection were at a much higher level above control values. In the first experimental block, D.B. scored 28/30. In the control block that followed immediately, in which all trials were 'blanks' but the switch was continued to be used, he scored 20/30. When, in the next block of all 'blank' trials, the switch was no longer operated, he scored 16/30. We then immediately gave another experimental block, with light vs. no light, and he scored 26/30. In other words, his performance with genuine stimuli was 28/30 + 26/30 = 90 per cent. The control for the switch artefact gave the same percentage score as in the other field, namely 67 per cent (and again without the switch the score dropped to chance at 16/30).

The next step was to test the form discrimination in the impaired field, and this was done in two further blocks. He scored 31/60 = 51.7 per cent. Finally, we returned to the good field with the form discrimination with one more block of trials, and he performed at 93.3 per cent (28/30). If all these results are assembled, as in Table 27, it will be seen that, again, there is double dissociation between the two fields and the two tasks. The good field yielded a 90 per cent score for form, and only 71 per cent for detection; the impaired field gave a score of 90 per cent for detection, but only 52 per cent for form.

Table 27   Double dissociations

	Triangle vs. cross	Grating detection
Left field — 18° 10′	14/30 + 15/30 = 29/60 = 48%	28/30 + 26/30 = 54/60 = 90%
Right field — 73°	27/30 = 90%	15/30 = 50%

	Curved vs. straight triangles	Spot detection
Left field — 80°	31/60 = 52%	54/60 = 90%
Right field — 80°	54/60 = 90%	64/90 = 71%

A final control procedure was run in the impaired field. It was interesting and important to see whether D.B. could actually detect the triangle in the impaired field, even though he could not discriminate its curvature. If he could not detect the presence or absence of the triangle, he presumably could not be expected to make the curvature discrimination. Therefore, he was given a further 90 trials at the same eccentricity (80°) in which half consisted of the straight triangle, and half of a blank white card, and asked to respond 'blank' or 'not blank'. He performed at 77/90 correct, or 85.6 per cent. Then, to ensure that he was in fact detecting the presence or absence of something on the card, he was given a discrimination between two blank cards, and he performed at chance, 30/60.

A paradox arises, of course, as to why the impaired field should actually possess apparently *better* sensitivity for the spot detection task than the normal field. There are two possible reasons. The first is that he might have adopted a different criterion in the two fields, not only in the technical sense (for which we have no firm evidence for or against) but also in the colloquial sense. Psychophysical determinations are tiring procedures for subjects as well as experimenters. We always gave D.B. the opportunity to rest between blocks, but were surprised how fresh he appeared to remain while testing of the impaired field was progressing, whereas he tired more normally for testing in the intact field. When questioned about this on one occasion, he said, 'But I am not *doing* anything in my blind field — I am just guessing'. On his intact field, he had the attitude of a very conscientious and intent subject.

There is, however, a second possible answer that lies in the sensory mode itself, namely that his right eye was found to be less sensitive than his left for detection (see Chapter 4) most likely because of the pupillary constriction associated with his right cervical sympathectomy. At an eccentricity of 80° on the horizontal meridian, only the ipsilateral eye has a visual field, i.e., stimuli fall in the monocular crescent. Therefore, at these extreme locations, the sensitivity of the impaired field would be governed entirely by the left eye, and that of the good field entirely by the right, less sensitive eye. We originally favoured the first explanation (cf. Weiskrantz 1980), before the calculations comparing the two eyes had been completed. But the explanation in terms of differential sensitivity of the two eyes now seems the more likely, because it is only at these extreme locations that we have ever found the impaired field to be clearly more sensitive than the intact field, whereas a criterion shift ought to apply more generally over the whole extent of the field defect. This matter was pursued in an experiment with an artificial pupil to check on this possibility, with results that support the view that the difference in pupil sizes of the two eyes accounted for their difference in sensitivity (see Chapter 11).

Whatever the explanation of this particular aspect of the second experiment it adds further support to the results of the first. In both situations, the impaired field had a bias in favour of detection in relation to the intact right half-field, which in turn had a bias, under the specific conditions of these experiments, in favour of form discrimination in relation to the field detect on the left. Therefore, it is reasonable to conclude that the two regions mediate qualitatively different types of visual function.

17 Standard situation

During the last few years of work with D.B., it became possible to test subjects with visual defects in a constant environment (space kindly made available by the National Hospital, Queen Square, London) and with a fixed procedure, so that a spectrum of capacities could be measured for comparative purposes. D.B. was tested on some of these procedures on three occasions, in September 1979, April 1982, and lastly in August 1983. The room was light-proofed, and surfaces that might be reflective were draped with black velvet. The front wall was covered with dark green hessian material, providing the tangent screen of $100° \times 100°$, with a subject sitting 1 metre from the fixation point in the centre of the screen. Eight Type Q3D projectors were positioned 2.44 metres from the screen, behind the subject, with two directed to each of the four quadrants of the screen. All stimuli for testing were presented by a projecting tachistoscope (Forth Instruments), consisting of a Kodak Carousel projector fitted with a beam interrupter in the focal plane, driven by an electronically timed solenoid. A zoom lens was fitted to adjust the size of each stimulus set precisely. The projector was situated 2.44 metres from the screen, on an adjustable elevated rack. The cover of the slide holder was opaque and in addition the projector itself was surrounded by an opaque case except for the front. Unless otherwise specified, the stronger of the two projector lamp settings was used, and the exposure duration of all stimuli except for movement was 150 msec. Only one quadrant was used for testing, with the two background projectors for that quadrant turned off, the other six remaining on. The background light level of the quadrant to be tested was -1.05 to -1.12 log ft lamberts. The level of the other three quadrants was 0.40 log ft lamberts. Only one standard position was tested, namely with the stimulus centered on a point 25° eccentric from fixation on the 45° off-horizontal meridian. With D.B. the quadrant tested was always the lower left or (for control comparisons) the lower right. The following sub-tests, time permitting, formed part of the profile: (a) flash detection threshold; (b) threshold for curved vs. straight triangles; (c) threshold for orientation discrimination; (d) figure-ground threshold, using dispersed or clustered material; (e) threshold for horizontal movement of a vertical line; (f) locating by reaching.

Unless otherwise specified, threshold determinations were derived from a modified staircase psychophysical method, using Gellerman random tables. The initial value was always placed at least three steps above the threshold estimated from pilot runs. If the subject scored six out of six correct, the task was made more difficult by one step. If a mistake occurred in the first group of six trials, the block was extended to 10 trials. If there were no more errors, the task was made more difficult by one step. If two errors occurred in a block of 10 trials, another block of 10 was given. If the subject scored four errors or less in the combined block of 20, the task was made more difficult by one step until he scored more than five errors in a block of 20 trials. The threshold was then defined as the interpolated 75 per cent value. The staircase was then moved up in reverse order to check on the value, and if there was a discrepancy of more than one step, the procedure was repeated. As was our policy, *no* knowledge of results was given during the course of any of the determinations.

The specific parameters used for each sub-test, together with D.B.'s results on the two sets of tests, were as follows:

(a) Flash detection

The stimulus was projected disc of light, 10° in diameter. A set of neutral density filters was mounted on a wheel placed in front of the projector lens, allowing attenuation from maximum intensity in steps of 0.1 log units, over a range from 0 to 3.9 log units. The light value of the disc at the 0 attenuation setting was 0.67 log ft lamberts. Because of the ambient level generated by the six other projectors illuminating the other three quadrants plus the general illumination provided by the projector, producing (as already mentioned) an ambient level on the test quadrant of -1.12 log ft lamberts, an attenuation of 1 log unit produces a light level of the projected disc of -0.3 log ft lamberts, two units of attenuation, -0.84 log ft lamberts, and three units of attenuation, -1.06 log ft lamberts.

The tolerable light level below which stray light artefacts could be safely ignored was assessed by having control subjects cover their right eye completely and mask the left half of their fields in the left eye with a black card. The attenuation at which the flashed disc presented at the standard position in the lower left quadrant, on a random Gellerman schedule, could no longer be detected at all was determined. The same procedure was carried out by shaping spectacle frames and goggles with close-fitting surrounds with the left half-fields masked out over the lenses. This tolerable value is less than 0.7 log units of attenuation (for this eccentricity of 25° along the 45° off-horizontal meridian). (If a dark foundation cream and face powder are placed on the nose, the safe level could be reduced to between 0.3 and 0.4 log units of attenuation.) Therefore, if any subject gives a threshold value of less than 0.7 log units of attenuation in this detection task, his score was rejected as being possibly due to diffusion of light. This was *not* a problem for D.B., whose threshold levels of attenuation at this locus in the field were much higher than the permitted lower limit.

The tachistoscope was operated on every trial, after a ready signal, but on the 'no-light' trials, the light path was blocked in front of the lens by an opaque card (well behind the subject). The subject was instructed to say, 'light' or 'no-light', and to guess if he could not see or was uncertain.

On the first occasion, in September 1979, D.B.'s threshold was 2.92 log ft lamberts of attenuation, and in April 1982, it was 2.95 log ft lamberts of attenuation, i.e., he could just detect the disc when it had a light value of just under -1.06 log ft lamberts (against a background of -1.12 log ft lamberts). On the third occasion, in August 1983, his threshold was slightly higher, 2.60 log units of attenuation (-0.97 log ft lamberts), but the ambient illumination was also slightly higher on this occasion, and the difference in threshold cannot be assumed to have any significance. Control subjects' thresholds have not been measured, but they are somewhere between 3 and 4 log units of attenuation. D.B. has a deficit, but it must be considered to be mild.

Verbal commentaries

When the stimulus was well above threshold, he said he 'was aware of something coming in, and then going away'. As the intensity decreased in the staircase procedure, he said, 'it is now coming in much slower'.

(b) Curved vs. straight triangles

Lantern slides were prepared of the series of outline triangles whose sides had varying degrees of curvature (previously described in Chapter 8). The centre of the equilateral triangle was at the standard position in the field. The bottom of the straight triangle was horizontal, and spanned 10° of visual angle. The series started with straight vs. the most curved (C-7), and proceeded in steps of one in the series. In 1979, D.B.'s threshold was 5.02, and in 1982 it was 5.62 (the higher the number the poorer the performance — control subjects can usually discriminate the hardest item in the set, no. 1, from the straight triangle at 90 per cent or better under these conditions). His performance must be considered to be poor.

Verbal commentaries

In 1979 he commented, 'waves were either sharp or not so sharp. I could recognize it as a triangle from the sharpness'. In 1982, he said of the easiest value, on which he did well, 'something came in every time, but I was just guessing about "straight" vs. "curved". No idea — just 50:50'. He said it was 'just the same as before' when he was judging the hardest value given to him (C-5), on which he performed at chance.

(c) Discrimination of orientation

The stimulus was a square wave grating within a circle of 10° diameter. The centre of the grating was at the standard position. The grating always had nine cycles across its diameter. The light value of the bright stripes in the grating was 0.8 log ft lamberts, and of the dark 0.0 log ft lamberts. A series of gratings were prepared with their orientations rotated off-horizontal in steps of 5°. The standard grating was always horizontal, and the alternative one non-horizontal, and the subject was asked to respond 'horizontal' or 'non-horizontal'. The first discrimination in the series was horizontal vs. vertical. If the subject succeeded at that, the next was horizontal vs. 45°. After that the step size was 10° until the subject first made an error, and thereafter 5°. In 1979, D.B.'s threshold was 10.0° off horizontal. In 1982, it was 13.12°, both below normal but nevertheless reasonably good.

Verbal commentaries

In 1982 after the horizontal vs. vertical values, on which he performed perfectly, he said, 'pure guess-work'. As the series proceeded, he said, 'about the same as before: 50:50 (chance).' No commentary is recorded for the 1979 test.

(d) Figure-ground, clustering

The rationale of this test was to determine how closely packed a dispersed set of small spots must come before they are identified as a 'figure' (although there are, of course, other interpretations that can be placed upon the test). At one extreme the stimulus was one in which they are closely packed in the shape of a circle. In the most dispersed stimulus the dots were spread out more or less randomly over the quadrant, with the constraint that they should have approximately equal packing in terms of visual angle at different eccentricities. The flux of all stimuli in the series was constant. (We are grateful to Miss Joyce Bolton for the tedious work involved in preparing the stimuli.) The centre of the closely packed distribution fell on the standard location in the field, and had a diameter of approximately 10°, but with some scattering within a diameter of 25° along the 45° lower left meridian. The discrimination always started with the easiest value. There were five steps between the dispersed and clustered extreme values, no. 6 being most dispersed, and no. 1 most clustered value (Fig. 29, 1–6). The discrimination was always between no. 6 as the standard and one of the other five. The subject was asked to respond 'clustered' or 'spread out'. In 1979, D.B. had a threshold of 2.5. In 1982 he performed rather better, and had a threshold value of 4.5. A control subject would be expected to be above threshold, but not perfect, with the most difficult value, no. 5, and therefore D.B.'s most recent score represents a relatively mild deficit.

Verbal commentaries

In 1979 he remarked, 'I said "clustered" when something like a pole was going into the wall. I was aware of nothing when I said "spread out"'. In

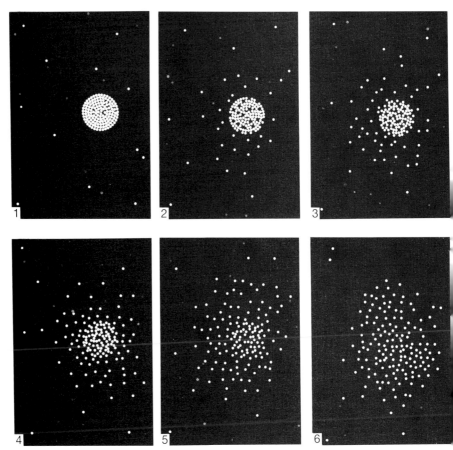

Fig. 29. 1 to 6. 'Figure-ground clustering' stimuli, from most clustered (1) to most dispersed (6), with centres of clustering presented at 25° eccentricity on 45° lower meridian for 150 msec. (See text for further details)

1982, he said that he responded 'clustered' when 'it was fast moving', and 'spread out' when it 'was slower moving'.

An additional 'figure-ground' test was also used in a preliminary way, based on 20 slides of varying signal to noise prepared by Warrington and Taylor (1973) for routine testing of patients. The letter 'O' was presented against a grid with varying densities of random small spots. In half the items the contrast was dark on light, and in the other half the opposite, so that the task could not be solved on the basis of flux alone. The series was graded in difficulty by varying the ratio of black to white in the figure in relation to the ration of black to white in the ground. Fourteen of the slides contained the figure, and six did not, and D.B. was asked to respond 'yes' or 'no' to indicate presence of the figure. The order was random and presented twice, the second in the reverse order. The centre of the 'O' fell at the standard locus in the field, and measured approximately 10° across the diagonal formed by the 45° meridian on which it was placed, and the duration was 150 msec. The task turns out to be too difficult for controls with these stimulus parameters; they score only about 75 per cent correct. When tested in 1979 D.B. scored 57/80 (71.2%) but on finer analysis he was better than 93 per cent on the eight easiest slides (30/32 correct). However, on another occasion in 1982 this was not confirmed. An improved version of the test for brief durations in eccentric vision would be very useful as it would measures of signal-to-noise detectability. As far as the results go, they suggest a moderate level of residual capacity for figure/ground organization. His verbal commentary, even when he was performing well on the easy stimuli was 'pure guess-work', 'not aware of any shape', 'no idea how well I did'.

(e) Threshold for movement

The set-up has been described above (Chapter 6). A vertical line, 10° in length, was projected by a mirror attached to a galvanometer, which was oscillated at adjustable rates and amplitudes linearly across the field. The centre of the line fell at the standard position, 25° eccentricity on the 45° lower left meridian. The frequency of the triangular control wave was set at 2.45, 5.39, 11.13, and 16.12 Hz, in that order. The reverse order was then presented. Each ascending and descending order was presented four times. At each frequency the amplitude of the excursion was gradually increased ('method of limits') until the subject responded. The threshold for each frequency was the average of the eight amplitudes at which the response occurred. The results of D.B.'s test on this procedure in September 1979 (the only occasion) have already been presented in Table 20. His verbal commentaries, in which he said he could not see the line or the light, but 'felt' the movement, are also described in that section.

(f) Reaching

Reaching for stimuli in the Aimark perimeter also formed part of the standard procedure, with positions among 6 positions presented in random order. The size, location, and brightness of the stimuli could be varied, depending on the sensitivity of the subject and the limits of the field defect, but in the standard version the target was the 1° 40′ stimulus, with a light reading of 1.18 log ft lamberts, against an ambient level of −1.65 log ft lamberts. All of the results for D.B., carried out both in the standard situation and in various other conditions, have been summarized in Chapter 3.

Part III

18 Review of other cases

Examples of residual vision in a field defect are not difficult to find. Clinically, all cases of 'relative' scotomata, as distinct from 'absolute' scotomata, by definition possess degraded vision rather than total and profound blindness within the field defect. These are Gordon Holmes's cases of putatively 'incomplete lesions' of visual cortex causing 'an amblyopia, colour vision being generally lost and white objects appearing indistinct, or only more potent stimuli, as abruptly moving objects, may excite sensations.' (1918, p. 361). The degree of 'incompleteness' would, according to writers such as Poppelreuter, determine the amount of uncovering of hierarchical layers of visual capacity that would occur, going from amorphous light sensitivity, to size perception without definite form, to amorphous form perception, to perception of discrete objects, to mild amyblyoia, to normal vision with decreasing severity (and possibly with complete recovery). Whether this hierarchy refers to degrees of severity or 'completeness' of lesions, to area 17 alone, *or* to area 17 *plus* surrounding cortex of areas 18 and 19, is, as we have reviewed, still unsettled (Chapter 1).

Rarer but more dramatic claims have been made for the loss of specific attributes or classes of attributes with otherwise relatively preserved vision. Cases of achromatopsia, for example, show selective loss of colour vision without corresponding loss of discrimination of achromatic features. Riddoch (1917) reported cases with loss of perception of static objects but relatively sensitive preservation of moving objects. Holmes tended to be sceptical of this and also of achromatopsia being specific defects beyond those that could be explained by amblyopia, and he used normal far peripheral vision as a kind of simulation of such defects (Holmes 1918, p. 379). In this he apears to have been too conservative. The recent well-documented case report of Zihl, von Cramon, and Mai (1983) (and the earlier related reports by Pötzl and Redlich 1911; Goldstein and Gelb 1918) of loss of movement perception, with intact perception of static objects, certainly cannot be explained in such a way, and of course would also fall outside Poppelreuter's hierarchy of degrees of fragility. At a 'higher' level are various forms of agnosia which display relative loss of specific categories of visual perception, such as prosopagnosia, topographagnosia, autotopagnosia, in which acuity and other dimensions of visual capacity may be quite intact. An exhaustive review of this interesting and important area is beyond the scope of this monograph, but fortunately neuropsychological reviews are available (cf. Bauer and Rubens 1985; Warrington 1985).

This section will be restricted to a much narrower class of cases, namely to clinical, demonstrable field defects within which certain attributes of visual capacity are unexpectedly present. By 'unexpectedly' one refers to the experienced clinician or to the patient, most commonly to both. Much turns, of course, upon the precise meaning of 'unexpectedly'. Standard clinical methods may not possess adequate sensitivity to reveal some amount of vision in a severe but nevertheless not absolute field defect. But the experienced clinician would not, nevertheless, be surprised in such a case if more searching methods revealed, say, an ability of a subject to respond to large and abrupt transitions between very bright light and absolute darkness, especially if the subject is dark-adapted, as in case already mentioned by Bender and Krieger (1951; cf. Chapter 1). If he followed up such a finding, he would then know pretty well what to expect in a range of demanding visual tests for such a patient who had just a modicum of sensitivity remaining, e.g., poor visual acuity, lack of form discrimination, reasonably intact movement perception for large stimuli, degraded colour vision, etc. What *would* surprise the experienced clinician, and the patient alike, would be if a 'blind' patient nevertheless showed a fine sensitivity and good discriminative capacity when tested under certain conditions, that is, if there were an unexpected discrepancy between a capacity revealed by some methods and by others. 'Blindsight' is perhaps the most extreme example of such a discrepancy; it refers to the situation where a patient shows a loss of awareness of any vision, or at best only a very degraded awareness, while at the same time displaying a sensitive capacity for detection and for performing certain discriminations that are independent of the requirement for acknowledging awareness, as we have seen with D.B.

Clinical methods — indeed, also laboratory methods — for testing human visual capacity implicitly and almost inevitably depend upon a verbal exchange in which the subject is asked to say 'whether' or 'what' he *sees*. It would be tedious in the extreme to proceed non-verbally. (In testing animals we are precluded from using such an expedient, which is one reason why animal psychophysical testing can be so tedious and lengthy.) But even if a 'non-verbal' response mode is used, such as a response key, the tester will nevertheless almost invariably instruct the subject to respond when or according to what he *sees*. The subject is tuned in to answering what has been called a 'commentary' type of question (Weiskrantz 1977), regardless of whether he actually answers it 'verbally' or 'non-verbally'. If he cannot acknowledge seeing but could nevertheless discriminate he would not respond by pressing the 'I see it' key. It may seem strange to consider how a visual discrimination could be made in the absence of 'seeing', but this is a question we will address more fully in the next chapter. The point to be made here is that the typical test of human visual capacity focuses the subject's attention directly and usually explicitly on his visual *experience*.

The more general point, however, is that an 'unexpected' revelation of a capacity may occur when one uses an unusual method of testing for it. But there is another way in which a difference between what is found and what is expected can arise, which derives from the stage at which the 'state of the art' has reached. A new discovery or an advance in knowledge may well be unexpected at first, but eventually — perhaps rapidly — becomes the predicted and perhaps even commonplace outcome, and is incorporated into a revised 'paradigm' (Kuhn 1962). No-one is now surprised by finding that monkeys without striate cortex, when tested by a methodology that gradually has become refined, can detect gratings and locate visual events in space. It was very surprising when first discovered, when the expectations were based on 'total luminous flux'. If 'blindsight', as revealed by forced-choice methodology, were commonly tested for and commonly found, it would no longer become unexpected.

It is too soon to say how common it will become. Quite aside from the inevitable slowness with which forced-choice testing itself can proceed, if a capacity such as that found with D.B. depends on a lesion being relatively restricted to area 17, then this is also bound to be far from common, let alone universal (see Chapter 1). But it is clear that forced-choice methodology by itself is not sufficient to reveal residual capacity in all 'blind' field defects caused by occipital cortical damage: some scotomata are determinedly absolute (Weiskrantz 1980), although one can never rule out the possibility that residual function might be revealed by other as yet undeveloped methods. Therefore, as far as the current 'state of the art' is concerned, it will generally be difficult for the clinician or researcher to predict in advance whether residual vision will be revealed in a scotoma classified as 'absolute' by conventional perimetry. But, of course, the individual patient can still be very surprised if one can demonstrate to him that he can discriminate in the absence of 'seeing'. A number of cases have been reported in the literature which bear varying degrees of similarity to D.B. This list does not claim to be exhaustive, but is reviewed to give some idea of the range of findings, and to see if any common threads emerge.

The fact that control of pupil size by light is retained (although depressed, Koerner and Teuber 1973) in patients with blindness caused by occipital lobe damage is proof enough of a separation between awareness and some effect of light on the brain (the reflex is known to be mediated by a pretectal pathway). Similarly, ter Braak *et al.* (1971) have reported preserved optokinetic nystagmus in a cortically blind patient (this optokinetic response is also reported to return in monkeys with striate cortex removal, Pasik and Pasik 1964). Both of these examples are of 'reflex responses' and as such may be denigrated to the status of isolated and low-level fragments not normally involved in discriminative function. But we are not, in any event, aware of them, whether we are normal or not, and they are not under our own control.

As already mentioned, one of the first explicit reports where the contrast was drawn between residual function involving voluntary control by stimuli in the apparently 'blind' field came from Pöppel *et al.* (1973). Four patients with occipital lesions (one vascular, three traumatic) were tested, all of whom had a region in their visual field in which there was 'no light perception', although in none was there a complete hemianopia. The subjects were required to move their eyes to the position at which a light (2°, 100 msec duration, 1 log unit above background intensity) had been projected in their blind field. 'As the patients had no light perception within their scotomata, they were not able to "see" the visual stimuli to which they had to respond'. Therefore they were told to 'guess' where it had been presented. Eye movements were recorded.

There was a weak but significant correlation between target position and eye movement angle for stimuli within 30° of the fixation. Two subjects with retinal scotomata were tested as controls for scattered light (also with a more intense light, 2 log units above background), and they showed no correlation. There was also a 'catch trials' control in which light stimuli were not actually presented in conjunction with the accompanying auditory signal, and this too yielded uncorrelated results. Pöppel *et al.* speculate that the eye movement control was mediated by some midbrain mechanism. As regards the subjective character of the blindness of the fields tested, they comment, 'it is interesting to note that the patients had no feeling about the presence or absence of light stimuli; actually they believed that their performance was always completely random'. (p. 296).

Very shortly after our report on D.B. the first of the studies from Lyons Laboratory appeared. Perenin and Jeannerod (1975) tested six adult patients with field defects caused by various lesions of the occipital lobes, and two control patients with pregeniculate lesions. Subjects had to identify a simple pattern flashed on a screen, either verbally or by selection from a multiple choice array. Then they were asked to point with their finger at the location where the flash had occurred, whilst still maintain fixation. The flash was quite intense, produced by a photo-flash (1.5 msec., 70 j). The results are not provided in detail, but it was reported that patterns could never be identified as such. But the flashes could be detected 'in most cases', although localized about one third of the time at the fixation point (this presumably due to diffusion of light); for the pregeniculate cases this was the *only* response. But the flash could also be localized within the 'blind' field by the occipital patients, who could point to its position 'with good accuracy'. Pregeniculate patients could not locate in their blind fields. Interestingly, in one subsidiary experiment an occipital patient who was not 'aware' of the existence of a pattern flashed into her 'blind' field, and could not locate it by pointing, nevertheless showed typical eye movements in the direction of the 'after-image', the pattern being that observed by normal subjects when they attempt to look at an extra-foveal after-image. This study suggested, thus, a preservation of ability to locate but no evidence of preservation of pattern discrimination.

The reports so far have all been of patients with posterior cerebral lesions involving mainly the occipital lobes. A most remarkable set of observations on a group of patients with cerebral hemidecortication has also been published by the Lyons group (Perenin 1978; Perenin and Jeannerod 1978). Six patients were studied in whom this extensive surgical procedure was carried out for treatment of infantile epilepsy and hemiplegia from various aetiologies. All of the neocortex and hippocampus and part or all of the caudate nucleus were said to have been removed, and in three cases there was histological confirmation of the ablated calcarine cortex. On perimetric examination all subjects had a homonymous hemianopia with partial sparing of the macular region from 2° to 6°. There were, in addition, two control subjects with pregeniculate chiasmatic damage that had caused a complete bitemporal hemianopia without macular sparing.

To assess spatial localization, stimuli (either spots of 2° or 3.5° diameter or a grating 6° × 8° with various exposures) were projected onto a hemispherical screen and subjects were required to point to the location with a stick held with a fully extended arm. The contrast between stimuli and background was moderately high (2.4 log unit difference from the grating and 2.7 for the spots). Both the intact and impaired half-fields were studied. 'On the hemianopic side, as [the subject] could not actually "see" any target, he was required to give a forced-choice response, i.e., to point to where he "guessed" the target had appeared'. (Perenin and Jeannerod 1978, p. 3). A clear and significant correlation between target location and pointing in the blind fields was found with each of the hemidecorticated subjects, although the relationship was not as strong as in the intact half-field. With the two control subjects, pointing responses in the blind half-fields were never found to be correlated with the target location.

Performance was somewhat improved when longer stimulus durations were used (100 to 500 msec), and also slightly with larger stimulus sizes, and with a moving rather than a stationary grating. In two subjects it was also noted that there was a good correlation between target location (100 msec duration) and the position to which the eye moved.

The subjective reports using these high contrast stimuli are of some interest. The controls reported a glare spreading out from the middle of the screen into the normal half-field. The hemidecorticated patients 'had the feeling that a quite bright light had been turned on in the impaired part of their visual field, and was spreading from there into the normal field. But none of the subjects could "see" the form or size of the target, nor have any conscious idea about its location, which they only "guessed" when required to respond in the tests'. (p. 4). 'Whether [subjects] may be aware of the existence of a stimulus within their "blind" field, or not, they have to use a "guessing mode" in order to give the required response'. (p. 9). Although there was obviously diffusion of light into the normal field under the conditions of this study, the authors dismiss its importance for localization because measured diffusion from the target from one half-field to the other hemifield was independent of stimulus locus, and of course the control subjects failed to localize the stimuli in their impaired half-fields, in contrast to the hemidecorticate cases, despite equivalent conditions of diffusion.

As in other group studies, there were some noteworthy individual differences among subjects. The most important factor in allowing better performance appears to have been the age of the subject at the time of the initial damage to visual cortex, although with this small group the evidence cannot be conclusive.

Perenin (1978) went on to examine pattern discrimination in these same subjects. Circles vs. triangles (solid or outline figures), and horizontal vs. vertical lines or dots were projected into the impaired field (with a difference of up to 2.84 log units between stimulus and background, duration 100 or 500 msec). Also, in one condition the stimulus/background contrast was reversed (log difference 0.30). Performance was not striking. Only two of the six patients showed a significant discriminative performance—the same two, as it happens, who were best in the localization tests—but the better of the two only scored at 72 per cent correct overall, and the poorer, just 57.2 per cent. Again, with the high contrast stimuli that were used, the reports of the subjects are of interest. Controls reported seeing 'a very dim light arising from the middle of the screen' when the stimulus was flashed in the impaired half-field, whereas 'hemidecorticated [subjects] felt a rather bright light arising from their impaired visual field. But none of the [subjects] could "see" the form of the pattern, which they had to "guess" when required to respond in the tests'. (p. 699). Again, for the same reasons as in the localization studies, together with the fact that reversing the stimulus/background contrast did not impair the performance, diffusion of light was discounted by the author.

Evidence of shape perception in a scotoma was also pursued by Barbur, Ruddock, and Waterfield (1980) in a carefully controlled psychophysical study of their 22 year-old subject 'G.' who had become blind in his right half-field after a road accident at the age of 8. G. is 'unable to detect or recognize objects located in the "blind" hemifield and regards himself as blind in the right half-field.' (p. 906). Barbur *et al.* found that under their conditions G. would detect flashed and moving targets, but with much less sensitivity than in his good half-field. With a circular light target of 1.2°, no detection was possible up to the maximum contrast level of 2.40 log units above background (except in a small region of foveal sparing already known to exist). But when the size was increased to 5°, detection was possible at any location in the impaired hemi-field *if* the target was flashed. 'If it is not flashed, he is unable to detect it . . . even if it is slowly translated at 2° per sec (p. 909). As the background luminance was increased, his increment threshold for flashed or rapidly moving stimuli (40° per sec) increased in the predicted manner, but the threshold values were some two log units greater than those for his normal half-field (and for other normal observers). The 'blind' hemifield had a low critical fusion frequency, large spatial summation, but a high sensitivity to fast moving targets. Velocity discrimination in the impaired field was normal, even though the shape or size of the target is not discriminated.

In order to see whether spatial localization was possible without 'awareness', Barbur *et al.* reduced the light value of the flashed stimulus (1.7° diameter) so that it was 0.5 log unit below his detection threshold (luminance value not given). A calibrated graticule was placed in the background field with which G. was made familiar, and he was then requested to state verbally the estimated calibration number on the graticule for flashed targets presented in random locations in the scotoma out to an eccentricity of 24°. G. showed evidence of good ability to localize the 'unseen' targets that had been flashed into his impaired field. He was more variable, but his mean values were quite similar to those of his good field.

Size, orientation, and shape discriminations were also examined, all at suprathreshold contrast levels of 0.75 log units (duration of 250 msec). Sizes of circular targets varied between 1.5° and 8.3°. When suprathreshold levels were equated, he was unable to discriminate. Discrimination of orientation (a 12° × 1.35° target placed in a vertical, horizontal, or 45° position) also yielded chance performance. Finally, identification of a circle, square, triangle, or rectangle, each of 6.6 degrees^2, was also at chance. Thus, G. showed a good ability to localize targets and to respond to fast moving targets in his impaired field. He could respond to flicker and to intensity increments of flashes, but with an impaired capacity. Shape and orientation seemed to be impossible, within the limits tested, even though the targets as such were above the threshold for detection. Unpublished evidence (Barbur, personal communication) also confirms that targets placed in his impaired field (2° diameter, 1.16 log units above background) can exercise a control over saccadic eye movements of appropriate amplitude, although with decreased accuracy and increased latency.

G.'s subjective experience suggests that he is not blind given a sufficient salient stimulus. If a target of sufficient size (more than 1.2° diameter) and intensity (2 log units more than the threshold for his good field) is *flashed*, he reports 'a dark shadow.' At higher intensity levels, 'it sometimes appears as a localized, bright flash' (Barbur *et al.* 1980, p. 910). The authors discount an explanation of these or any of their other findings in terms of scattered light.

More recently Ruddock and his colleagues (Blythe *et al.* 1985, and personal communication) have extended their methods to a study of a population of 25 subjects with 'blind' scotomata caused by cortical damage. In 5 subjects (including G.) they found evidence of residual function for flashed or moving lights within the field defect, as well as an ability to locate the stimuli by hand-reaching or by eye movements. As with G. originally, the subjects cannot recognize or discriminate the pattern of targets within their field defects. They again examined and rejected an explanation of their positive findings in terms of light scatter.

Cases with bilateral occipital damage resulting in a defect over the entire visual field would make assessment of residual function easier because the need to maintain careful fixation and control for stray light artefacts would be circumvented. Such cases without additional extensive damage are rare, although the two cases of Brindley, Gautier-Smith, and Lewin (1969) show that even here there is some crude detection of light onset and offset (see Chapter 1). But a bilateral case deliberately studied in the context of blindsight research, using forced-choice methods, has been reported by Perenin, Ruel, and Hécaen (1980). The patient had a dense ischemic lesion of both calcarine cortices (as seen on CT scan). He showed some capacity to localize flickering, but not stationary, lights even though he 'did not really see them'. Moving stimuli often produced 'seeing' responses although 'he could not tell at all what it was that was moving or gave curious responses.' (p. 610). The authors conclude that they were 'able to demonstrate the reappearance of some visual capacities, even though the patient still behaved as if completely blind in everyday life and the lesion remained as it was first seen'. (p. 612).

Another single case study of a patient with a very large, but not complete, bilateral scotoma was reported by Bridgeman and Staggs (1982); perimetry (target and luminance conditions not described) revealed only a small area of intact vision about 9° in radius in the right hemifield, with some macular sparing. The visual defect was caused by bilateral subdural hematomas resulting from a blow to the occipital lobes in a traffic accident. The subject was instructed to move a pointer to the estimated position of a target stimulus while maintaining fixation (with eye position monitored). The subject was first trained with a high contrast target (3.87 log units), a triangular patch of white light 2° wide × 3° high. In the first condition, the target oscillated slightly in the horizontal plane. Then, still using the oscillating target, contrast was reduced to 3.01 log units. Then further sessions were given with a stationary target. Finally, the oscillating target was used with a low contrast (0.66 log units) target. There were also control sessions in which no target was actually projected on the screen.

The results were that relatively poor localization was found at the beginning of the first session, but performance gradually improved with practice (the subject received no feedback about errors). By the end of the training with low contrast target his performance was good across the whole field, although apparently somewhat better in the right than the left side of the scotoma. There was a clear monotonic relationship between target eccentricity and pointing response across the scotoma from positions 15° to 45°. Performance during the control trials was clearly uncorrelated with target position. The authors' principal concern was to demonstrate 'plasticity', improvement with practice to a level that was quite creditable: by the final day with the low contrast stimulus, there was a monotonic relationship between target eccentricity and pointing. They also remark that this showed some transfer to everyday natural conditions: 'following the extensive practice with simple targets, the subject reported an improved ability to recognize movement within the scotomas, giving him an ability to sense approaching objects when walking and reducing his anxiety in crowds'. (p. 1202).

Not much attention is given to the subject's own commentaries. It is said that he eventually could 'recognize movement' and 'sense approaching objects'. It is also said that he 'reported receiving more information about position at the off-transient with fixed targets (but not with oscillating ones)', but this is followed immediately by the comment that 'the subject could not discriminate control trials from experimental trials'. (p. 1203). It is not clear how these various statements hang together, although it is possible that the last comment refers only to the oscillating trials.

The group that has, more than any other, focused on recovery of visual function with practice is Zihl, von Cramon, and colleagues at the Max Planck Institute in Munich. Their work is also relevant to the response modes that might be available in the absence of awareness. They distinguish between improvement with practice in 'blindsight', without any change in field size, and recovery leading to enlargement of the visual fields, which they suggest has a different basis. Here we shall review the salient features of their findings in both categories, although we shall leave the question of their interpretation to a later stage.

All of the field defects studied by Zihl and colleagues were measured in the Tübinger perimeter. Under most conditions a 116′ detection stimulus was used with a contrast of 2 log units above background for dynamic perimetry. For static perimetry, this was also the maximum contrast. It is important to note that their *target* stimuli for localization or other tests of residual function typically have a lower contrast level (usually by 1 log unit) than the stimuli used to plot the scotomata, against the same level of background luminance and in the same apparatus, and so evidence of any residual capacity, when it occurs, is in response to a weaker stimulus than that which yielded zero sensitivity in perimetry in the same region of the scotoma.

Two of their studies are directed to the question of whether some autonomic features of the 'orienting reaction' might be detectable in response to light, and further whether other non-verbal motor responses might have 'access' to visual stimuli presented in a field defect. In the first of these studies (Zihl, Tretter, and Singer 1980), the electrodermal skin response was measured in response to moving stimuli briefly presented well within the scotomata of two patients, assessed as blind with dynamic and static perimetry in the Tübinger perimeter (with a maximum intensity of 320 cd/m^2). The light stimuli (32 cd/m^2 with background of 3.2 cd/m^2, $2°$ diameter, 200 msec duration) 'moved between about $30°$ to about $45°$ eccentricity along the horizontal axis, since we observed that stationary stimuli were less effective in eliciting this electrodermal response'. The stimulus and 'blank' trials (equal numbers, randomly arranged) were each preceded by a click. Skin conductance was measured on the surface of the left hand for every trial. There was a greater number of electrodermal responses to light trials than to blanks, a highly significant result. The responses to light trials were also significantly larger in amplitude. It is also of some interest that the conditioned eyelid response to light was found to be intact in monkeys with complete removal of striate cortex (Marquis and Hilgard 1937).

In a related study (Zihl and von Cramon 1980), three subjects with large but incomplete hemianopias (resulting from surgical removal of abscess, trauma, and embolism) were tested for their detection of stimuli (116′ diameter, 1 log unit contrast, 100 msec) flashed in the field defect. Three response modes were studied separately: voluntary blink; key press; or a verbal 'yes' response whenever they 'felt' that a light stimulus was present. The patients, on the basis of the density of their scotomata, were said to be 'obviously without any conscious visual access'. Finally, localization within the field was measured by instructing subjects to shift their eyes to where they guessed the target had been presented. The subjects were given several testing sessions over two to three weeks, and were never given knowledge of results.

In the first session performance was poor on all measures, but with practice they improved and by the last session their ability to indicate the presence of a light target by blinking or key-pressing markedly improved after a few hundred trials, 'even though they never reported seeing a light target'. (p. 291). Statistically the results were significant for all three patients. In contrast, their verbal responses to lights vs. 'blanks' was random and insignificant. They were not given extended practice with the localization of targets but after their practice sessions with the detection task, their localization accuracy was also seen to have improved and their saccadic responses were highly correlated with target position.

As both the key-presses and the eye-blinks were voluntary responses, it is curious that these response modes were able to reveal a clear discrimination between lights and blanks, whereas the verbal response 'yes' did not. A subject might be persuaded to 'guess' 'yes' just as readily as to press a key. The answer perhaps lies in the meaning of the different response modes to the subjects. If, as the authors argue, they had 'no conscious access' to the lights, a 'yes' response verbally produced might have interpreted by them to mean literally 'yes, I actually *saw* the light'. Whatever the explanation, the evidence is clear both for a residual sensitivity to stimuli well below the threshold for conscious detection under their conditions, and for its improvement (without reinforcement) with practice.

Another study by Zihl (1980) concentrates on the effects of practice specifically on localization by saccadic eye movements. Three patients with large scotomata (in one, bilateral in extent), due to embolism, haemorrhage and infarction were tested with the same stimuli as above (116′ diameter spot, 1 log unit contrast, 100 msec) placed randomly at positions between 10° and 45° eccentricity in the scotoma or, in other sessions, in the good field. Control sessions were also run in which 'blank' trials were given in which all other conditions were the same as the target trials. The patients were tested usually three times a week for three to five weeks, and were not informed about the results of the training sessions.

All three subjects' localizations were poor in the first session, but by the final session had improved, in one case to an almost perfect correspondence between target and eye position. The control trials in all three cases yielded, as appropriate, no correlated relationship. It is interesting that the saccadic latency was shorter to light stimuli presented in the blind hemifield than in the intact hemifield. There was no change in the size or density of the scotomata measured after the completion of practice sessions.

It is said that the subjects 'never reported seeing any targets during the test periods', although it is also commented that 'after a few hundreds of trials two patients were sometimes able to "feel" the correspondence between target and eye position'.

A more recent study by Zihl and Werth (1984*b*) reveals an important aspect of the role of practice: they noted that early in testing patients (again, with the same stimulus parameters as above) tend to make a constant saccadic sweep to stimuli in the scotoma, even though they have been told that the stimuli will vary in position from trial to trial. Subjects thought they were changing the extent of their saccades, but actually were not. Two (out of three) patients were then given feedback about the extent of variation of their saccades (but *not* about the accuracy) and encouraged to shift their final eye position if they did not do so in a block of trials. Needless to say, with a constant and unchanging saccade amplitude no correspondence between target position and eye position is possible. These two patients showed clear and impressive accuracy after this regime and with further practice (again, without feedback as to their accuracy). The third patient, for whom no such encouragement was given to break any fixation bias, eventually developed accurate saccades, but required more than 1000 trials to do so. The possible relevance and importance of this kind of factor in the uncovering of localization capacity in the blind field is obvious. It is suggested that patients with large field defects may develop eye movement patterns with respect to their scotomata which are rigid and unsuited to the specific demands of the experimental procedures needed to test for localization, and 'it seems a prerequisite for the patient's ability to use his localization capacity that his response mode is "shaped" so that he chooses frequently between various locations.' (p. 20).

The role of practice, especially as its benefits can be seen in the absence of direct knowledge of results, seems to lie not in practice with the particular responses as such, but in the attentional and attitudinal mode with which he responds. It is claimed, in this connexion, as we have noted, that practice with a detection task *per se* will transfer to saccadic localization without further practice (Zihl and von Cramon 1980).

Zihl and Werth (1984a) also carried out a searching study for the possible influence of stray light on saccadic localization, a question that has been of concern to all investigators in the field. Their strategy was deliberately to introduce stray light from the target by increasing its contrast level. Two patients with scotomata, both caused by pseudocystic necrosis of the visual cortex or radiations, had field defects assessed in their standard perimeter, with a target 2 log units above background (which was $3.2 \, cd/m^2$). Static perimetry was also carried out up to a maximum of 2 log units above background. Saccadic eye movements to a flashed target were then investigated, with the targets presented either at $10°$, $20°$, $30°$, and $40°$ eccentrically, or in one experiment, either at $5°$ and $30°$. As usual, there were 'blank' control trials.

The patients were first tested with a 'low' contrast level, target level 1 log unit above the background level of $3.2 \, cd/m^2$ (duration 100 msec). Both patients showed good localization with saccadic eye movements to the guessed position of the flashed target, one of them in the first session, the other after two sessions. Under this low contrast condition, the authors stress that 'neither patient reported any awareness of light or visual sensation in any trial. They described their responses as guesses. This means that the amount of stray-light emitted from the target never produced the sensation of light, even when the target was presented at $10°$ eccentricity. In fact, the amount of stray light measured under this condition hardly exceeded the background luminance.' (p. 5).

When the subjects were then tested under a very high contrast level of 4 log units (target $320 \, cd/m^2$, background $0.03 \, cd/m^2$), the results were quite different: the subjects were at chance. Both patients reported a diffuse light appearing in the intact part of their fields. The patients still pointed to the impaired field, but 'both . . . were convinced that the light always must have been presented at about the same location, because they were never aware of any difference with regard to the "size" or brightness of this diffuse light.' (p. 7).

The same results were obtained with a 2 log unit contrast level (target 320, background $3.2 \, c/m^2$), i.e., chance performance for localization. The same was also true even after another 720 trials of practice with the high contrast target, and also when just two target positions instead of four were used. Finally, when contrast was again reduced to the 1 log unit level for one patient, performance again was very accurate. Stray light, therefore, strong enough to be detected by the subjects, actually interfered with good performance, the important implications of which we shall be taking up again in the next chapter.

In these studies by the Munich Max Planck group, the size and density of the scotomata typically did not change as a function of practice, although the subjects' localization or detection by 'guessing' did improve. This rigidity of the field defect contrasts with other findings by the same group in which some scotomata could be made to contract with practice.

In their most recent paper (Zihl and von Cramon 1985), the results of training on some 55 patients with scotomata of varying aetiologies are reviewed (a few of whom, however, were also included in an earlier similar study, Zihl 1981). In effect, the training procedure was closely similar to the 'practice' method in their 'blindsight' studies. The patient was instructed to move his eyes to the 'guessed' position of a briefly flashed target, either 1 sec or 100 msec; this appears not to be an important parameter in allowing recovery to occur (Zihl 1981) even though in the 100 msec condition the stimulus cannot be captured by an eye movement, given the longer latency period of a saccade. (In an earlier study by Zihl and von Cramon in 1979, repeated determinations of detection thresholds were used instead of eye movements as the training method, and this method also was effective.) Targets were presented at different random positions between 10° and 40° eccentricity, depending on the perimetric details. Training sessions of 80–120 trials were given at least three times a week, or daily. Various details of the area of intact vision were measured, including form, colour, and acuity. It was found that in about 80 per cent of their patients there was some enlargement of the visual fields. In about half of these cases, the increase was not large — 5° or less (although when this occurs near the fovea this can be clinically very useful). A quarter of the cases, however, showed increases ranging from 10° to 48°. The important point is that in most of their patients the newly recovered part of the field included form and colour perception, and from this the authors conclude, reasonably, that in such cases there must have been striate cortex surrounding the remaining field defect that had not been irreversibly damaged.

The analysis of their cases suggests that recovery of form and colour is less likely to occur in cases of closed head injury than in cases of vascular accidents. They also conclude that treatment is not likely to be effective in those cases where there is complete necrosis of cortical tissue, as judged to exist when the CT scan showed hypodense lesions with values of less than 15 HU. Finally, the gradient of sensitivity between the intact and 'blind' field appears to predict, although not with complete certainty, whether training will be effective in enlarging the field of vision. Where the gradient is 'shallow', i.e., gradual, rather than sharp, training is more likely to be effective. The gradient must be judged, however, against the statistical effect of eccentricity itself, because it tends to be more shallow the greater the eccentricity. Shallowness of gradient is of interest in relation to animal work because the field defect caused by a lesion of striate cortex in the monkey produces a shallow gradient (Cowey 1967). Indeed, the gradient is, by definition, 'shallow' because sensitivity is still present with a target that is both smaller in size and of lower contrast than one which produces zero sensitivity in the scotomata of Zihl and colleagues' patients.

The question of recovery in relation to 'blindsight' will be returned to in the next chapter, but here it is useful to point out that the method used to demonstrate residual function, with a possible potential for gradual improvement with training, is precisely the same one as that which may yield a shrinkage of the field defect with training. And so a distinction between the two outcomes is based not on methodology, but on whether one is concentrating, on the one hand, on the residual function that can still be found even in a scotoma which is absolutely dense in perimetry, or, on the other hand, on the recovered sensitivity that is seen in the enlarged field of vision as the scotoma shrinks. Whether different or common mechanisms is involved is quite a separate issue.

Detection within the 'blind' field involves the same methodological issues as in any psychophysical detection task, but the relevant signal detection methodology has rarely been applied in the testing of residual function. A carefully conducted recent exception is the study by Stoerig, Hübner, and Pöppel (1985), who plotted the ROC (receive-operating-characteristic) curves for a patient at three positions in his scotomata, plus the optic disc 'blind spot' within the scotoma. An ROC curve is a plot of 'hit rate' against 'false alarm rate'. The patient had an incomplete left hemianopia caused by an infarction of the right occipital lobe two years prior to the study. His field was plotted perimetrically with a target of the same parameters as the Munich group, namely, a 320 cd/m^2, 116' target against a background of 3.2 cd/m^2; both dynamic and static perimetry were carried out.

For the test itself, the target was smaller — only 44' — and the luminance was just 1 log unit above the 3.2 cd/m^2 background. Its duration was 200 msec. To obtain ROC curves, blocks of trials were given in which the ratio of target-on to target-off trials was varied between 20:80 and 80:20. The results were clear: significantly positive discrimination was found at the three positions in the scotoma, but at the optic disc — as with D.B., in a study with the same aim — the subject was at chance. The results are obviously relevant to the issue of scattered light. The subjective lack of awareness of the patient is described strikingly and unambiguously: 'Over and over again he claimed that he had no sensation whatsoever, that he was only guessing, and could hardly believe that his performance was above chance'. The authors go on, 'we conclude that he had access to some information mediated by the blind field, and from his statements we conclude that he did not have any conscious perception. In this sense it can be said that he was unaware of his performance'. The paper includes a useful and concise analysis of possible mechanisms that might be involved in mediating residual visual capacities.

Thus far all the studies we have reviewed have focused rather directly on the control of responses by visual targets within the impaired field, principally on localization as inferred from eye movement shifts or by pointing, or on detection as revealed either verbally or non-verbally. But by now a variety of other approaches have been invented. At this stage of development of the field, such a variety is to be applauded rather than condemned. It will be from a convergence of methods that fuller understanding and increased practical control will emerge. All of the studies to be reviewed next include the interactions or comparisons, implicit or explicit, between the good and impaired field.

The same patients tested by Pöppel *et al.* were also included in a study by Whitman Richards (1973) within a larger group of patients in whom the possibility was examined that there might be some retention of stereoscopic capacity in the field defect. The details of his procedures and results are heavily compressed in tabular form and are not easy to reconstruct; it is clear that quite exacting arrangements would be needed to replicate his situation in detail. He found that stereo discriminations were absent or greatly impaired when light bars (0.82 log units above background light level, 80 msec duration) were presented entirely within the scotoma. However, surprisingly, patients could discriminate above chance as to whether a monocular or a binocular stimulus was delivered to the blind field. If one of the two stimuli was presented just inside the intact field, and the other to the blind field, the discrimination was better. The performance improved still further when dark bars on a light ground were used instead of light bars on a dark ground — a test introduced to control for diffusion of light — even when both bars were in the blind field. Indeed, they may be better discriminated in the scotoma than in the intact portion of the visual field. Richards also included one control subject with optic nerve damage (and with higher contrast stimuli), with appropriately negative results. It is also clear that not all patients were equally proficient at the monocular/binocular discrimination.

Richards's comments that 'when the flashes were presented to the blind region, nothing was reported seen, so he was forced to guess. At first, the subjects were reluctant to make guesses about something not seen, but eventually they could be persuaded to go along with the eccentric request'. (p. 335). He did note, however, that there were some conscious sensations under certain conditions with some (but not all) of the subjects, but even when these occurred, they were non-veridical: 'flashed contours appear instead as scintillations, pin-pricks, needles or small flashes such as "gunfire at a distance". Such sensations occur only for light flashes'. Dark bars (for which performance was better) did not yield such experiences. He summarizes his findings as follows: 'In contrast with other animals, when the occipital cortex is damaged in man, blindness occurs in spite of intact retinal projections to subcortical centres in the midbrain. By a proper selection of stimuli and responses, however, it can be shown that some information about the visual stimulus may be processed in regions of cortical blindness, even though the stimulus is "not seen". . . . The nature of the residual discrimination has the properties of a primitive stereoscopic mechanism that ignores the sign of the stimulus disparity.' (p. 333). (Although not directly relevant to 'blindsight' as such, the report by Ruddock and Waterfield (1978) is of another interesting example of stereo perception in the absence of pattern perception. They investigated a subject who could not perceive images formed with light at the 'red' end of the spectrum. He could nevertheless construct stereo images formed by a fusion of red and green array of random elements, although he could not perceive the elements of the red pattern.)

A somewhat similar idea was used in an elegantly simple approach by Marzi *et al.* (1985). They exploited the fact that the reaction time to two flashes presented simultaneously to a normal subject is consistently faster than the reaction time to a single flash, whether or not the two flashes appear in the same hemifield or whether they appear in opposite fields. The rationale was, thus, to see whether this held true for patients when one of the two stimuli fell within the blind hemifield, even though it is 'not consciously perceived'. The stimuli were 'small LEDs'. They found that some, but not all, hemianopic subjects (8 out of 11) tested showed a trend towards faster reaction times when the two flashes were presented across the vertical meridian, even though the subjects reported seeing only one stimulus—the one in the intact field. 'In two further patients there were convincing signs of blindsight when they were tested with a low intensity flash in the intact side and a brighter flash in the blind field'. As this report appears only in abstract form more details are awaited, but the approach would seem to hold considerable promise as a simple and readily available technique.

The link between extra-striate pathways and 'attention' is one that has long attracted interest and given impetus by 'two visual-system' speculation. A rather neat approach to this problem was developed by Singer, Zihl, and Pöppel (1977). They measured detection thresholds in normal subjects at varying eccentricities for targets presented in the Tübinger perimeter (either of 27′ or 116′ diameter, 500 msec duration). They found that with repeated determinations at the same locus, a subject's sensitivity typically declined by 0.2–0.3 log units. (Their paper actually reads 0.5–1 log unit, but this is a mistaken reading from their scale [personal communication]. We have confirmed the 0.2–0.3 log units result. It does appear to be important, to obtain the effect, to have variable inter-stimulus intervals, not a fixed interval. This detail is not in the published paper, but is confirmed by personal communication with the authors). Such adaptation occurs more readily with peripheral than central targets, and the adapted field is somewhat larger than the adapting target itself, reaching a diameter of 20° in the periphery.

An important feature of the adaptation, or desensitization, is that it can be reversed quickly, in one of two ways. If a mirror symmetric region of the other half-field is adapted in turn, the sensitivity of the original position recovers, is 'reset'. Or, if a saccadic eye movement is directed towards a target in the mirror symmetric half-field, the original sensitivity is also reset. The resetting does not occur if the saccade occurs in the absence of a target in the mirror symmetric half-field, or if the 'resetting' target lies outside a mirror symmetric field. Now, having determined these relationships in normal subjects, these workers went on to report that the 'resetting' target, i.e., the one that returns the original sensitivity to its original strength after adaptation, can be a signal that occurs within a 'blind' scotoma. 'Although the patient could not see the stimuli, he was asked to pay attention to any events which might be perceivable in his blind hemifield. The appearance of the light stimuli were signalled to the patient by the noise of the shutter system. Since there were no responses from the patient the same sequence of stimuli was repeated which had caused adaptation in his intact hemifield. Immediately after this adapting procedure in the blind hemifield, which lasted 30 seconds, detection thresholds in the previously adapted area within the intact hemifield were measured and found to be reset to control values.' (p. 181). They report, further, that such a procedure was ineffective if the target was not in the mirror symmetric region. Finally, as the link with midbrain mechanisms was of prime concern, they studied a patient with a retino-tectal lesion, and indicated that no resetting of thresholds occurred in that case.

This view of a reciprocal interaction between mirror-symmetric regions of the fields as they project on the superior colliculus is suggested not only by the animal lesion evidence (Sprague 1966) and electrophysiology (Goodale 1973) but also by the report by Pöppel and Richards (1974) of two patients with 'double' scotomata. Both patients had extensive field defects in one half of the visual field together with small scotomata in the opposite visual field. In both cases islands of increased sensitivity within the large scotoma could be found corresponding to the mirror-symmetric locations of the small scotomata in the other half-field, supporting the concept of a loss of inhibition as suggested by Sprague (1966).

Various reports have appeared of completion of figures in or across the 'blind' field (e.g., Poppelreuter 1917; Warrington 1962), but these have typically involved stimulus situations where, in fact, the 'filling-in' would not be veridical, i.e., the subject treats an incomplete figure as though it were actually presented as a complete figure; Warrington's findings strongly suggest that the lesions of the parietal lobe are likely to be involved when this occurs. A somewhat different approach involving 'veridical' completion was employed by Torjussen on subjects with field defects (1976, 1978; cf. also Bender and Teuber 1946 for a similar suggestion). If an incomplete circle was shown in the good field, subjects correctly reported it as a half-circle. Similarly, if a half-circle were presented within the hemianopic field, nothing was reported, i.e., it was not seen. But, if a complete circle was shown (Fig. 30), subjects reported a complete circle, even though half of it fell within the field defect and even though the subject was blind to half-circle alone

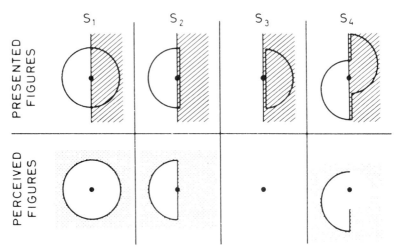

Fig. 30. Stimuli presented to blind (hatched) and sighted fields, with resulting perceptions by subjects in Torjussen's experiments. Dot in centre indicates fixation point. Scale: radius of circle is 10°. (From Torjussen 1976, by permission)

	Subject 1		Subject 2		Subject 3	
S_1 / S_2	◐	◖	◐	◖	◐	◖
○	97.5	5.0	92.5	6.7	89.2	5.8
◖	0.0	88.8	6.7	92.5	6.7	93.3

Fig. 31. Results of Torjussen's experiments with three subjects, showing per cent of responses of full or half-circles for stimulus conditions S_1 and S_2 of Fig. 30. (From Torjussen 1976, by permission)

in the field defect. The symmetry of the stimuli in the two half-fields was found to be important. If the half-circle in the blind field was displaced vertically from the one in the intact field, completion was not full.

   These results were obtained on three subjects (Fig. 31) for whom not many clinical details are provided, nor are perimetric details available beyond the description of having been plotted with a Gambs perimeter. All three had 'macula sparing 3°.' In one study the stimuli were exposed briefly with a photo-flash, inducing a crisp after-image a few seconds after the flash. The after-image was 'viewed' against a large flickering background, and the after-image persisted for several minutes. The same stimuli were used in a separate study with the same subjects, but presented tachistoscopically, up to a maximum of three seconds, until a recognition threshold was attained, but the actual durations are not reported. The contrast was low — a maximum of 0.62 log units above a background of 5.6 log ft lamberts. The results were substantially the same with both modes of stimulus presentation. The results might seem to be complicated by the macular sparing, but this could not be the explanation of why stimulus condition S_1 did not produce the same perceived response as S_4 (Fig. 30). Also, the stimulus presented to the blind field alone was horizontally displaced from the vertical meridian into the blind field. The tachistoscopic procedure would avoid light scatter, given the low contrasts, and eye movements or biased fixation should have yielded different results than those obtained for S_1 vs. S_3. Unfortunately, Torjussen was unable to continue this line of clinical research, and it would be useful to follow up this promising approach more systematically and with a wider range of patients with more clinical detail. Marcel (personal communication) states that he has confirmed the essential features of Torjussen's findings in two cases and extended it by varying the distance of the stimuli from the vertical meridian. Another related positive confirmation has been reported by Perenin *et al.* (1985).

Another type of 'veridical completion' (Ruddock, Waterfield, and Barbur personal communication) showing interaction between the good and 'blind' fields emerged from manipulating the parts of the figure that generate 'illusory' Kaniza triangles (cf. Gregory 1972). The procedure is to place two of the corners in the good field, angled so as to suggest two of the corners of a triangle. In the blind field the third corner is placed either correctly aligned, or aligned inappropriately for generation of the illusory triangle. The subject is asked to respond simply, 'triangle' or 'no triangle' (Fig. 32a,b). Patient G. of Ruddock and colleagues (Barbur *et al.*, 1980; see above, p. 122) was able

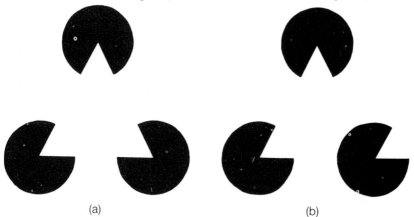

(a)   (b)

Fig. 32. (a) 'Regular' and (b) 'irregular' imaginary Kaniza triangles. Subject is asked to respond 'triangle' or 'no triangle'. Critical part of the display, the lower right circle with cut-out, is presented to the 'blind' field. (By courtesy of Ruddock, Waterfield, and Barbur)

to perform this task, even though he could not 'see' the critical portion of the array located in the field defect. I (unpublished, brief mention in Weiskrantz 1980, p. 378) have been able to confirm this phenomenon in another subject, using Ruddock *et al.*'s stimulus material. She performed well above chance, to her surprise when shown her results. Marcel (personal communication) has also confirmed this in two subjects using the Kaniza figures.

A different example of interaction can be seen in a recent study by Pizzamiglio, Antonucci, and Francia (1984). They exploited a phenomenon described for normal subjects by Dichgans *et al.* (1972). If a large disc, covered by random dots, is rotated in front of a subject, it produces a sensation of body rotation in the opposite direction; there is also a shifting of the apparent vertical in the opposite direction, and cyclotorsion of the eyes in the same direction as the rotation. Pizzamiglio *et al.* showed that a smaller effect is found with a rotating disc presented to just one half-field. They then argued, reasonably, that if a rotation within the whole field produces no greater after-effect than rotation of the good half-field alone, it can be inferred that the blind field does not contribute to the induced after-effect. Also, if there is residual vision, the rotating display within the field defect should produce an effect in the expected direction (tilting of the vertical in the direction of rotation).

They tested seven patients with complete homonymous hemianopias resulting from vascular lesions. Their stimulus display was a large disc, 120° of field, covered with black 3° spots, rotated for 2 min. Half-field stimulation was produced by masking half of the display with a white screen. The subjects could adjust a line in the middle of the display to his subjective vertical before and after rotation of the disc.

It was reported that in all seven patients there was positive evidence of a contribution of the 'blind' field to the adjustment of the vertical as seen by the good field. In each case the subjective tilt produced by stimulation of the good field was greater than stimulation of the normal hemifield alone, and the effect was approximately the same size as seen in normal subjects. The effect of presenting the disc to the blind field alone was small, but in the predicted direction. The authors speak against an artefact due to involuntary eye movements during testing, and also said that 'none of the patients exposed to visual rotation in the blind-field was aware of anything happening on this side. Only [one] patient commented that she "could not see anything really moving on the right side", but from time to time, she has the impression that "something, not clearly definable, was happening on the right side"'. On the other hand, the half-field stimulation had a curvilinear border (to prevent the screen being used as a vertical frame of reference) and it seems that stimulation of the blind half-field may have intruded slightly into the good half-field, even though the after-effect is strongest when induced with peripheral field stimulation.

For this reason it would be useful to test controls subjects with pregeniculate damage and also to vary the conditions of half-field masking. But the technique is elegantly simple and potentially well-adapted to use in the clinical setting. It may also turn out to be a more sensitive indicator than other methods: as the authors comment, 'although the number of subjects is not sufficiently large to make generalizations, the difference between entire vs. normal hemifield stimulation was observed in all cases and in almost every trial. These results may be due to either the specific sensory nature of the task, which may be more sensitive to visual blindsight, or to the different response paradigm which, in our study, requires the patient to continuously adjust a "visible" target instead of "guessing" or verbally describing brief stimuli' (p. 97).

Marcel (1983*a*,*b*) has taken the question of blindsight to a much higher level of processing which would necessarily involve detecting properties of shapes and also of semantic meaning. He studied the adjustments that his two subjects (one of them was G., studied by Barbur *et al.* 1980, see above, p. 122) made with their hands when reaching for objects in their field defects, and noted that they were appropriate to the shape and disposition of the objects. Even more surprisingly, if words were flashed into the field defects, meaning could be conveyed even though the words were not 'seen'. This was assessed by giving them subjects a choice of words in their intact fields immediately afterwards and asking them to guess which of the two was related semantically. These remarkable results are not yet published in full, and so the methodological details cannot be assessed, but the findings are rather similar to those that emerge from the domain of 'subception' and involve capacities that go beyond any others reported for blindsight. It remains to be seen how common such capacities will be found to be in other patients, using Marcel's methods.

Many, if not all, sensory modes share with vision the capacity both to detect and to identify the sources of their stimulation. Multiple parallel routes are also a feature of many sensory systems. The case reported by Paillard, Michel, and Stelmach (1983) of a dissociation similar to those we have been reviewing, but in the tactile mode, is therefore of considerable interest. The patient had a left parietal lobe defect which resulted in a severe tactile anaesthesia of the right side of her body. She failed to respond to touch of her right arm, 'even to the strongest pressure'. But when asked to point (blindfolded) to where she was touched with the pressure instrument on her 'unfeeling' arm, she was able to point, 'to her own considerable surprise', to the approximate locus of stimulation, although not as accurately as a control subject. The patient's comment (but in French) was 'but I don't understand that! You put something here. I don't feel anything and yet I go there with my finger . . . How does that happen?' Also contrary to expectation, she did react positively to moving stimuli on her arm and could judge its direction. She also showed some improvement in detection with practice in subsequent sessions. The parallel with visual residual capacity in blindsight is drawn explicitly by the authors.

As an autonomic electrodermal response has been observed to visual stimuli in the absence of 'seeing', it is of interest that a similar dissociation has been reported at a 'higher' level of visual processing. Travel and Damasio (1985) showed that two prosopaganosic patients who failed to recognize familiar faces verbally nevertheless displayed a clear and strong skin conductance response to photographs of familiar faces relative to control faces.

Finally, one must consider negative reports. In the nature of the situation investigators will not find it easy to publish failures to find a phenomenon. Quite aside from pressures upon journal space, very few workers are sanguine about trying to bolster the universal negative. But some negative reports have appeared, most notably by Campion, Latto, and Smith (1983). They tested three subjects. No clinical details are provided for two of the subjects, except that they, like the third, had homonymous hemianopias. In the course of their experiments, one subject died, and another was not tested further because she was 'less reliable in her fixation and performance, and had unstable fields'. Their best subject for their purposes was a 'young, well motivated, and co-operative' patient whose 'surgical notes indicated total removal of the left occipital pole'. Their observations led them to conclude that light scattering into the good field was sufficient to produce 'blindsight', and they went on deliberately to demonstrate that light scatter in normal subjects (themselves) could be used as a cue for carrying out discriminations such as localization, orientation, and detection. On the basis of their observations, plus a review of the literature, these authors did, indeed, lean heavily and somewhat tendentiously towards the universal negative. Fortunately, all of the workers whose work was reviewed had an opportunity to reply, although not given the final word.

That 'commentary' issue also included one report of a failure to find visual field increases using the methods of Zihl and his collaborators, without however providing any essential details. But, as Zihl and von Cramon themselves insist, the issue of recovery of function with retraining in areas that had been, but are no longer, in the field defect is separate from the question of residual function within the scotoma itself. The potential benefits of retraining are sufficiently important that it seems clear that further work will be pursued to see if human subjects' field defects can be made to shrink with retraining in a manner analogous to that seen in the monkey, and as with many other issues in the field this is a matter for future research rather than premature foreclosure.

General questions, both methodological and theoretical, that arise in connection with studies in this field will be discussed in the next chapter, as well as comparisons with our results with D.B. Here, assuming that the findings of these other studies are genuine, i.e., not based on artefact or deception, either by or on the investigators, what are the overall conclusions to be drawn from these studies?

First, if by 'blind' field we mean one in which the subject reports having no visual experience, then all investigators included in the review (except for Campion *et al.*) have reported some measure of residual function in the areas of 'blindness' caused by cortical damage.

Second, this does not mean that all fields tested were 'blind' under all conditions, i.e., never yielded reports of visual experiences, or were blind over the whole extent of the field defect. In many cases this *was* true under all conditions, but sometimes with high contrast or particular types of visual stimuli subjects reported experiences such as 'dark shadows' (Barbur *et al.* 1980), or 'pinpricks of light' (Richards 1973), or 'light arising from the impaired half-field' (Perenin). In some instances, abnormal patterns of detection of experienced visual stimuli were reported, e.g., the abnormally low c.f.f. for patient G. (Barbur *et al.*).

Third, evidence of residual function in the absence of acknowledged awareness measured in relation only to stimuli *wholly confined to the field defect* is largely restricted to: (i) detectability, whether by verbal report or non-verbal measures (many authors) and (ii) spatial localization, as revealed either by eye movements or pointing (many authors). In some instances, detection occurred more sensitively to moving or flashed stimuli (Barbur *et al.*). When specifically sought, evidence for shape discrimination was either absent (Barbur *et al.*), or weak (Perenin 1978), and the same was true in both of these studies for orientation discrimination in the frontal plane.

Fourth, evidence was richer and more varied when interactions between the 'blind' and intact fields were examined. Thus: (i) not only could detection *per se* be inferred from reaction times to one vs. two stimuli bridging the intact and blind fields (Marzi *et al.* 1985) but there is also evidence of (ii) monocular vs. binocular discrimination, (iii) perception of figures part of which appear in the intact field (Torjussen 1976, 1978; Barbur, personal communication), (iv) 'resetting' of depressed sensitivity following adaptation in the intact field by stimulation of a mirror-symmetric region of the blind field (Singer *et al.* 1977), (v) tilt after-effect induced by rotating stimuli in the frontal plane (Pizzamiglio *et al.* 1984), and (vi) semantic processing of words in the blind field affecting choice of words in the intact field (Marcel 1983*b*).

Fifth, the cases are by no means uniform, although as we have seen there are certain common threads. However, it certainly is not to be expected that brain pathology will be homogeneous in a region where several visual areas, striate as well as visual 'association' cortex (i.e., pre- and peri-striate) are compressed (see Chapter 1). Single case studies may be more revealing than group studies, at least until the picture becomes clearer with good grounds for selection of cases. But the richness in diversity clearly has positive benefits because of the potential for uncovering dissociations and can be welcomed on that basis (cf. Weiskrantz 1980).

Sixth, all authors have addressed issues of possible methodological artefacts either in their original articles or in response to critical reviews, among them stray light, intra-ocular diffusion, and inadvertent eye movements or faulty fixation. The issues will arise again in the next chapter, but here it is important to note the universal concern that the investigators themselves have had for adequate controls. It is not to be expected that every single study will contain the whole range of necessary controls, but it is clear from a number of studies, especially those involving the optic disc as a control, the use of low contrast stimuli, or the deliberate introduction of stray light, that the findings of residual function cannot be dismissed as artefactual.

Seventh, as yet no firm conclusions can be drawn very readily from any of the reports about the extent of the lesions or the critical structures involved in mediating residual function. The only studies involving *prima facie* complete removal of striate cortex plus extra-striate tissue are those of the Lyons group (Perenin and Jeannerod) of hemidecorticated subjects. No patients of any of the studies reviewed have yet come to post mortem. Again, we will return to this question of critical anatomical pathways in the next chapter.

Eighth, the field of evidence at this stage is still one in which a variety of approaches and interests is involved. There is not, as yet, a 'standard' methodology, either because work is at too early a stage of development or because particular workers have focused upon particular concerns. For example, only the Max Planck group (Zihl and collaborators) have concentrated upon the effects of practice and retraining. The richness of approach is one that means that new methods are still likely to emerge for some time, depending upon theoretical or practical concerns.

It is clear, however, that whatever interpretation one places upon mechanism or procedures, evidence for residual function in field defects has been produced that was not expected either from well-conducted perimetric charting with large, high contrast targets (thereby producing conservative estimates of size and density of the scotomata), from clinical reports, or from the experience of the subjects themselves. Depending on the continuing development of testing methods, imaging techniques, and the focusing of research interest, the question of whether residual function will turn out to be common, as suggested by Pizzamiglio *et al.* (1984) or seen only in a minority of scotomata caused by post-geniculate lesions, as suggested by others (Marzi *et al.* 1985; Blythe *et al.* 1985), will no doubt be resolved.

19   Status, issues, and implications

(a) Residual vision: description and comparisons

Leaving aside for the moment the question of D.B.'s verbal commentaries, and restricting ourselves to the objectively determined capacities, we can summarize D.B.'s discriminative skills as follows: He can detect and locate stimuli in his impaired field by pointing or, less well, by eye movements.

He appears to be differentially sensitive to detection *per se* as compared to shape discrimination, in contrast to his performance in the intact, normal half-field. He can discriminate the orientation of a grating in the frontal plane, with an accuracy that is surprisingly good (a difference of about 10° at a position 45° distant from the fixation point, which is approximately his capacity at that eccentricity in his good half-field). He can discriminate movement from stationary stimuli. Detection does not appear to be based on a special sensitivity to transient onset or offset properties of the stimulus events, because he can discriminate presence vs. absence even with a very slow rise time. His detection of a grating allows one, by varying spatial frequency, to measure his visual acuity; it is inferior to that of the intact field but quite creditable (2.6 cycles/degree at 30° eccentricity). His ability to discriminate orientation may be the basis of his skill in discriminating simple shapes, such as **X** vs. **O**, because he is poor at distinguishing between squares and rectangles matched in flux and also at other discriminations in which orientation differences are small or non-existent. On the other hand, he is excellent at discriminating squares from rectangles, where the principal cue is orientation.

Importantly, his visual acuity was *worse* with stimuli near the vertical meridian (15°) than slightly farther out at 25°–30° along the horizontal meridian, which would be difficult to explain on the basis of stray light or stray saccades to the good field. Earlier measurements along the horizontal meridian, prior to scotoma contraction, suggested that psychophysical gradients in general were reversed along the whole extent of the meridian, i.e., that he became increasingly sensitive with increasing eccentricity within limits imposed by retinal grain, just the opposite to that of intact vision, and this was taken to support the view that there was a bias towards peripheral vision (Weiskrantz 1978). However, measurements taken along the 45° lower meridian through the impaired field, after his scotoma had contracted to occupy mainly the lower left quadrant, showed that in general there was a decrease in these various capacities with increasing eccentricity in the field, as in the normal field, at least beyond 15° of eccentricity. On the other hand, along the 30° meridian, there was still the reversed gradient for detection (see Chapter 4). Thus, in retrospect, it seems likely that the reversed gradient, when found, may have been a reflection of using a meridian that did not run through the middle of the least sensitive area of the field defect. Of course, with perimetry it would have been impossible to determine this, and to have carried out forced-choice threshold determinations that completely mapped different meridia at a range of eccentricities would have been a daunting task. The inference here is based upon the fact that the regions of increased sensitivity were nearest to the part of the field that subsequently showed recovery. However, even along the 45° meridian, his movement threshold was poorer at 15° than at 25° eccentricity, obviously speaking against a stray light or stray saccade interpretation.

As regards his ability to compare stimuli either within or between his fields, it was noteworthy that he was *unable* to succeed in a 'same-different' task for two simple stimuli (**X** or **O**) when they were both *within* the field defect, at least under the conditions tested. He was well able to discriminate an **X** from an **O** within the field defect when presented singly. The same-different discrimination was an extremely simple task to perform using the intact field. As regards comparisons *between* fields, he was able to make a 'same–different' judgement between a form in the impaired field and another symmetrically located in the intact field. But as he could discriminate **X** from **O** in the field defect, it is not clear whether the matching between impaired and intact fields was based on a successive discrimination within each field separately.

For those tasks on which D.B. can be compared with other patients, his capacities are not markedly different. Other patients also are reported to demonstrate an ability to localize and to detect. His capacity to discriminate orientation is somewhat better than the other cases studied, e.g., G. (Barbur *et al.* 1980) and the hemidecorticated cases of Perenin and Jeannerod (1978; Perenin 1978), although neither of these groups of investigators used the same type of stimulus material as we did. It is not possible to make any confident statement about how well D.B. might do on tasks used by other experimenters but not yet tried with him, e.g., the Torjussen completion task, Kaniza triangles, double vs. single stimulation, after-effect of rotating stimuli. Nor have all of our procedures been pursued by others, e.g. matching within the field defect, slow stimulus onset, acuity, etc.). Indeed, one outcome of a monograph such as this might be to produce a greater future convergence. On the other hand, findings that go beyond what D.B. has so far been found to be capable of are those of Marcel (1983*b*), reporting semantic priming by verbal material projected into the blind field. D.B.'s shape discrimination would seem too weak for such processing. However, this is a matter of intuition rather than demonstration. Marcel (1983*a,b*) has reported that semantic features may be preferentially processed in relation to graphemic features for stimuli of which normal subjects are not aware (in a visual masking paradigm), and he links such observations directly to blindsight phenomena. And so the matter must be regarded as still open (see also below).

D.B.'s capacities are also not out of line with those reported for the monkey without striate cortex. Such animals can also locate stimuli in space, although (again, like D.B.) not with the accuracy of controls. They can discriminate differences in orientation of the same order of magnitude (8°, Pasik and Pasik 1980) as D.B. (10°). They can perform simple shape discriminations, although with some considerable difficulty. Their eye movements also can be controlled by targets in the blind field. They also have a reduced but creditable visual acuity of about 11 cycles/degree, but as the lesions were bilateral and the animals were presumably using their fovea, a direct comparison with D.B.'s acuity is not possible, and of course other parameters, such as contrast, were different. D.B.'s acuity (also reduced by approximately 2 octaves at 16.5° eccentricity) is within reasonable limits of an extrapolation from the animal results. All of these comparative psychophysical results with D.B., moreover, were obtained only when the forced-choice, 'non-verbal' methods of animal experimentation were employed.

Such is a blandly descriptive account of the residual capacities of D.B.'s field defect, and some comparisons with other patients and experimental animals. If the matter were to stop there, it would still be of considerable interest, given the history of this field of neurology, and comfort would be derived (for those who seek evolutionary continuities rather than dis-continuities) from the similarity with the results of animal research. But, of course, the matter does not stop there — it might even be said to begin there — given that D.B. is not a non-speaking, non-communicating creature. He can give his own reports of the situation and offer commentaries on the stimulus arrays. There are also implications for the understanding of the organization of the visual pathways themselves as well as the neurology of our ability to offer 'commentaries' on our discriminative performance, i.e., on the neurology of 'awareness'.

But, first, there are two other important questions to consider. The first is the question of validity: is D.B. somehow using his intact visual field to discriminate stimuli projected into his scotoma? That is, have we (including him) been deceived, unwittingly, by stray light reflecting around the room or diffusing within the eye itself? The second question is whether the properties of residual vision are like those of normal vision, but quantitatively degraded, or whether they are qualitatively distinct from normal vision.

(b) Stray light and other possible artefacts

It is impossible to prove the universal negative: it always remains possible that what appears to be a genuine discrimination may be based on a cue or cues that inadvertently intruded, and of which both subject and experimenter may be unaware. One can never exclude it absolutely, but only accumulate evidence that makes such a possibility extremely unlikely.

If 'residual' vision were not actually 'residual' in the impaired field but were based, instead, upon the use of the intact visual field, then obviously there would be no interest in the matter whatever. The issue that has most concerned virtually all the experimenters in the area of research, as well as some commentators, is whether discriminable light energy may have reached a preserved portion of the visual field, either through reflections in the room or through the media of the eye itself. The controls that other investigators have made have been outlined in the review of other cases in Chapter 18. As regards D.B., in our very early observations, control of conditions was far from ideal: no laboratory was available in the hospital in which light levels or other features could be carefully controlled, and light measurements were not made. It will be recalled that the very first observations of reaching were made in a quasi-bedside manner, under conditions of relatively strong illumination (fluorescent lighting) using 'naturalistic' stimuli, such as objects placed on the wall, the experimenters' hands, sticks, and the like, from which spread of light from objects into the intact field could hardly be a problem. It was D.B.'s positive responses to these that led to the use of the Aimark perimeter for a more formal reaching test, but at the outset no light measures were made; background conditions were low and the contrast was moderately high. D.B. and we were able to determine that there was no detectable spread of light on to the part of the perimeter arc projecting to the good field. Indeed, D.B. was very punctilious, then as always, in reporting to us if he detected any such spread of light into the good field, even if it was just a vague edge of a halo and of very weak intensity. As he remarked in response to an interview after he had successfully 'guessed' (to his great surprise) the various orientations of a stick in his 'blind' field under normal quite bright overhead illumination of the hospital setting, and was asked if he could ever 'see' the stick: 'No. That would be cheating *myself*'.

Of course, there *may* have been some cues in the room that he could use without his direct knowledge. And no doubt, one could so arrange cues deliberately such that stray light could be exploited by 'cheating', as Campion *et al.* did (1983), but as the early relatively informal conditions used by us with D.B. cannot be reproduced exactly in the absence of luminosity measurements and the use of a variety of rooms and a variety of conditions, further speculation about them is fruitless. Later tests were deliberately designed to overcome any such difficulties, and were specifically directed to the question of stray light. In addition, there were other observations on D.B. that seem to exhaust any possible explanation (of which we have been able to think) in terms of stray light or intra-ocular diffusion.

One way to control stray light is to make the illumination in the intact field so high that any stray light, even if it occurs, will be indiscriminable and undetectable. This was done both with the Aimark perimeter as well as another perimeter. The results have been reviewed for localization responses (Chapter 3). The level of ambient light was generated by using powerful photoflood lamps against which stray light from the perimeter target would have been insignificant, and the luminance and target size values used in these two experiments fall well within the limits advanced by Wilson (1968) for non-detectability of stray light into a functional field of vision.

A more tedious but very convincing test came from using the natural blindspot as a control for detection. Using forced-choice methods and a Latin square design, a small light projected onto the disc yielded chance performance—confirming that there was no discriminable diffusion with that target beyond 2° of arc. But when the light was projected on to areas of the scotoma neighbouring the disc, D.B. performed at well above chance using exactly the same forced-choice paradigm. These other loci are much farther from the edge of the intact field (itself plotted under conditions deliberately biased towards enlarging the intact field) than the same size spot is from the edge of the optic disc. If the light did not spread discriminably outside the optic disc, it is difficult to see how it could have spread outside the scotoma into the intact field from any of the loci in which it was placed. It is difficult to see how these results can be explained in terms of diffusion of light either within the eye or in the external environment, although for reasons that are totally incomprehensible to us, Campion *et al.* actually conclude rather perversely that this test provides 'very strong evidence *against* blindsight'. (1983, p. 478).

The natural blindspot was also used by Stoerig *et al.* (1985) in a signal detection test as a control for targets that were detectable in the scotoma. Other authors have employed control subjects with scotomata caused by pregeniculate lesions, or have shown that when stray light was deliberately introduced from the target into the intact field (Zihl and Werth 1984a) of patients with postgeniculate scotomata, or when eye patching was used to produce 'artificial hemianopias' in normal subjects (Perenin and Jeannerod 1983), spatial localization of targets in the 'blind' field was not found, i.e., there was not a discriminable basis for localization from stray light, even if present. All of these efforts, while they can never prove the universal negative, do very seriously diminish any claim for a definite positive artefact due to stray light.

There are also other test results with D.B. that would be difficult to explain as having been caused by a stray light artefact. It was possible to measure visual acuity within D.B.'s scotoma using sine wave gratings, and it is not easy to see how there could have been relatively undegraded diffusion into the good field so as to allow us to obtain a measure of minimal separable acuity on such a basis. Similarly, in our determinations of thresholds for orientation discrimination, the position and flux of a grating were held constant under all conditions — the *only* variable was the actual orientation of the stripes in the grating. And yet D.B. was able, by forced-choice discrimination, to distinguish a difference in orientation ('horizontal' vs. 'non-horizontal') of the order of 10°. Again, credulity would be severely strained to explain such findings in terms of stray light.

Another candidate for an artefact is faulty eye fixation or inadvertent, unmonitored saccades. Controls for this were deliberately introduced with D.B. Continuous eye movement recordings were made during one series of tests of reaching (Fig. 20), and indicated clearly that his fixation was well maintained (in fact, he was remarkably stable whenever we made such observations) and that his reaching responses could not be accounted for in that way. In another series of tests, we used short stimulus exposures (100 msec), a duration that is shorter than the latency for generation of a saccade, again without any degradation of his reaching responses (Fig. 19). That particular test, as it happens, was observed by a large number of colleagues in attendance. As a minimum of two observers were present throughout *all* of the tests with D.B., observation of eye movements could frequently be monitored, and the stability of his eye fixation and head position were excellent. In the 'standard situation' all durations were too brief to be accounted for in terms of inadvertent saccades, as was also the case for critical form discrimination tests and all of the matching within- and between-field tests. In the perimeter a chin rest, but no bite bar, was used, but head movements were not observed and would have had to have been extreme to have caused artefacts. Finally, the measured position of the optic disc for each eye provides a good indication of stability of head and eye position (and also of the possible occurrence of a pseudo-fovea, i.e., a constant shift in fixation to a non-foveal locus). The locations for the left eye and right eye were precisely where they should have been.

Again, other authors have used short durations and eye position monitoring to control for artefact. Advocacy of bite bars bears some flavour of obsessionality, and their absence can hardly account for the size of effects obtained in reaching and discrimination experiments in the blindsight literature. They may have some relevance, however, when relatively small effects are reported, e.g., when a small shrinkage of the visual fields is obtained, although to the extent that these effects are comparable to those found in the monkey, any such explanation would be highly unlikely.

While misleading or 'false' results due to stimulation of the *intact* field of view seem not to be an important possibility, there is one feature of D.B.'s field defect that could complicate some of the tests of reaching for randomly located stimuli. For some stimuli in some locations of the field, D.B. has a subjective feeling in response to a stimuli, e.g., of a localized 'something' moving in towards him; these reactions, which he denied were 'seeing', seemed to become more prevalent over the ten-year period. There was also an impression of 'waves' in certain regions of the field. These responses, when they occurred, were not uniform or present over the whole of the impaired field; in effect, this could mean that the various reaching responses were not independent, because if a 'feeling' did not occur to a stimulus after the warning signal, it could be assigned to a null region by a process of exclusion. Whether this occurred or not we have no direct evidence, but it increases the importance of those stimulus conditions in which 'waves' or any other subjective responses were quite absent if one wishes to avoid inferences that may have been made by D.B. based on such non-uniform properties of the impaired field.

(c) Degraded normal vision?

Having summarized the observed discriminative capacities above, one is naturally led to ask whether those capacities are qualitatively like those of the normal half-field of vision, but quantitatively weaker. But this question is, in fact, more complex than might appear at first sight, because the capacities of normal vision vary depending upon the position in the visual field, the adaptation level, and upon the physical characteristics of the stimuli themselves. It is, however, even more complicated than that: it is possible that, as stimuli in the normal field of vision become degraded, the qualitative profile of capacities of the visual system itself changes.

At one time we thought that the visual capacity of the monkey without striate cortex was like that of the normal peripheral visual field (Weiskrantz 1972): acuity, form, and colour vision are reduced, and detection remains reasonably intact. It also appeared in early (but not later) tests with D.B. that psychophysical gradients showed a paradoxical improvement in sensitivity with increasing eccentricity, just opposite to that of the intact field. The periphery can also be thought of as 'ambient' vision, with an alerting or attention-directing function, and hence would be quite consonant with a 'two visual system' approach (see Introduction and below). To the extent that D.B. can be used for forming inferences about this issue, however, the hypothesis of an equivalence to peripheral vision does not gain support.

Firstly, the evidence for a double dissociation between form and detection in two experiments strongly suggests a qualitative difference between his intact and the impaired fields. Second, in those same experiments performance of the intact field itself was assessed for points in the far periphery (80° in one test, 73° in the other, see Chapter 16), and therefore normal peripheral vision has qualitatively different properties from those of his impaired field, either in a peripheral locus (80°) or more centrally (18°). Third, on a number of occasions we presented a variety of stimuli to the far periphery of D.B.'s intact field and asked him whether they ever produced the quality of or had any other resemblance to any subjective experiences he had in his impaired field. The outcome was always quite firmly negative, and he remarked, 'No, even way out there in that part of my field, I *see*'.

The results of the experiments yielding a double dissociation between form and detection also rule out any simple explanation in terms of degraded visual acuity, because the detection stimulus in one such experiment was a sine wave grating and hence was supra-threshold for acuity. At a position in the field defect at which the grating could be detected highly reliably (lines vs. no lines), form discrimination was severely impaired. Conversely, at a position in the good field at which the grating could no longer be detected, the same form discrimination could be performed. And, again, the qualitative difference between the 'seeing' field and the scotoma was reported as being very clear by D.B. Thus, in the spared amblyopic crescent in the left half-field, while vision was fuzzy, he nevertheless reported it as *vision*. Measured visual acuity was, in fact, poorer in that region of the field than it was in the scotoma (which was measured at a less eccentric location than the amblyopic crescent), but despite this the subjective experience in the crescent was reported to be definitely and unambiguously of 'seeing', in contrast to the scotoma, where he said he was not even aware of the bright back-projected display within which the grating was generated (See Chapter 2). It has been claimed that the amblyopic acuity was actually better than that of the scotoma given that a different psychophysical procedure was used (Campion *et al.* 1983), but this lacks credibility (see below). In any event, a simple degradation of visual acuity can scarcely account for the properties of D.B.'s residual vision.

Similarly, any simplistic view that residual vision is dependent upon scotopic rather than photopic adaptation levels or mechanisms is inadequate, although animal spectral sensitivity evidence does suggest a shift to a larger rod over cone contribution after striate cortex removal in the monkey (Malmo 1966; Lepore *et al.* 1975). Spectral sensitivity has not been measured for D.B., or any other blindsight patient, to our knowledge. But at least some of D.B.'s capacities are present under photopic levels when rod mechanisms would be expected to be totally saturated. Thus, in order to eliminate 'waves', we used high levels of ambient illumination, and obtained good evidence of orientation discrimination. Visual acuity, also, was measured under photopic conditions, as were some of the **X** vs. **O** and movement discrimination tests which yielded positive evidence of residual function.

There is another type of degradation of normal vision that occurs in everyday life as well as under laboratory conditions, namely when a signal is too brief or too weak (in intensity, in contrast, or by masking) to enable readily acknowledged identification or even detection to occur, but which nevertheless may influence choice behaviour. This takes us into the field of 'subception' and to procedures such as backward visual masking. Typically one would expect forced-choice performance to be relatively unimpressive in response to a stimulus degraded in this way to the shadowy penumbra of the threshold zone, although it might be above chance. Thus, when we measured detection (presence/absence of a spot) in D.B.'s intact field at a far peripheral location (80°), he said he did not see the light. With forced-choice guessing, however, he scored at 21/30 and 20/30 correct, scores that are above chance (but still sub-threshold). But they are well below the 90 to 100 per cent performance that D.B. can display with a variety of stimuli in his field defect which he also reports not seeing: there are several examples, e.g., square vs. diamond, 95 per cent correct in 40 trials, with report of no experience of any kind, 'Nothing there. All guess-work'. (see Chapters 8 and 13). Such striking discrepancies between scores in one mode (square or diamond?) and the mode of reported experience (which can be defined as 'see' or 'not see'?) are not, in general, characteristic of responses to weak stimuli in the border area of near threshold determinations, where performance levels tend themselves to be marginal.

However, this is not always the case. In particular, Marcel (1983*a*) has reported a striking discrepancy, using a backward masking paradigm, between subjects' decisions when they had to report 'presence-absence' of a masked sample word, and another decision task, namely which of two visible words the masked sample word was graphically similar to, or, in yet another condition, which of two words the masked sample word was semantically similar to. The parameter in all three tasks was the interval between the

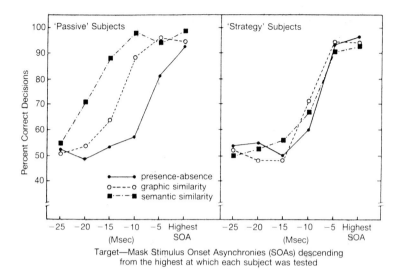

Fig. 33. Results of Marcel (1983*a*) with visual masking, showing per cent correct decisions with different types of stimulus content as a function of masking interval, for 'passive' and non-passive ('strategy') subjects. See text for further details. (Reproduced by permission)

stimulus and the masking stimulus that followed (adjusted for each subject separately). As can be seen in Fig. 33, left panel, subjects performed at 90 per cent in the semantic similarity judgement while their detection scores were at chance (50%), i.e., they could not discriminate on average whether a word was present, but could nevertheless base a semantic judgement upon it when it was.

It was on a closely related type of task that Marcel has found two 'blindsight' patients who also showed success, as we have noted (Marcel 1983*b*). That is, the subjects could not say whether a word (20 msec duration) was 'present' in their blind fields, but the interpretation of an auditorily presented polysemous word (bank) nevertheless could be biased depending on the meaning of the unseen word (river or money).

And so the question must be considered whether blindsight patients similarly, are, responding to visual events that are degraded by neurological damage such that the stimuli are below threshold for acknowledged detection but are nevertheless not completely blocked for other modes of processing. This is a serious possibility, but it does carry some paradoxical implications, at least as far as comparison with Marcel's findings is concerned. Marcel finds, counter-intuitively, and counter to any implication that blindsight is merely a normal response to an input with degraded informational content, that semantic information is the most resistant to degraded performance with masking, followed by lesser resistance of graphemic information, and that detection is the most readily upset by masking. In other words, the effect of masking is not an effect merely upon the *amount* of stimulus information. He argues (Marcel 1983*b*), indeed, for a qualitative dissociation of processing modes between 'non-conscious' and conscious events. Therefore, if blindsight were similar to the effects of background central masking in a normal subject, it would follow that patients would be able to perform quite high-level semantic and lexical decision tasks in the absence of any acknowledgement whatever that they could detect words. This may well turn out to be the case, as in fact Marcel has claimed for two patients. While this would have certain implications against an interpretation of blindsight as a response to 'mere' stimulus degradation, it would have even more remarkable implications for a quite large informational capacity of residual function in field defects of which the subject himself and the clinician alike would be unaware.

On the other hand, D.B. *was* able to carry out detection (forced-choice yes/no) under certain conditions, and yet his form discrimination was rudimentary and, we have argued, was possibly not even 'form' but derived from a capacity to discriminate orientation. And so, as far as the evidence goes, it would suggest a hierarchy opposite to that found by Marcel for masking. There may, perhaps, be one important difference of procedure and instruction. Marcel's subjects may not have been forced to guess about the presence/absence decision, especially as they had been first run through a threshold experiment for setting the masking time-interval limits. That is, they have been responding on the basis of 'see' or 'not see'. In contrast, D.B. was required for guess 'present' or 'absent' even when he did not 'see', and his behaviour was measured not only for his percentage of correct responses in forced-choice, but his verbal commentary was sought as well. Hence, in the detection task (see Chapter 4) for a briefly presented disc at 45° eccentricity, he performed by guessing 29 correct out of 30 and 18 out of 18, but remarked on questioning, 'just guessing. I don't think I did very well'. 'just guessing all the way through'. 'no idea'. On the other hand, it is possible that Marcel's subjects were more ready to 'guess' about the meaning or shape of the word. It would have been interesting to have had separate accounts not only of the subjects' decisions but their verbal commentaries as well.

If the human evidence has any direct link with the animal evidence, Marcel's masking results would be puzzling on that count. Monkeys without striate cortex can detect and locate visual stimuli; they also have a measurable minimal separable visual acuity and can discriminate orientation in the frontal plane. Their shape discrimination is less secure. Most important, however, is that the *meaning* of visual stimuli is erased, as described by Luciani originally and clearly elucidated by Humphrey (see Chapter 1). They can, for example, locate and retrieve fine and low contrast stimuli with exquisite dexterity, but cannot judge in advance whether the speck they are about to pick up is food or non-food. If they were strictly comparable with Marcel's subjects in terms of the preserved hierarchy of capacities, they might be expected to preserve their visual semantics (in the sense of the associations of reward or aversion with visual stimuli), but it is the disjunction between detection of a stimulus in the absence of recognition of its meaning that is such a striking feature of the destriated monkey. However, it is the counter-intuitive aspects of Marcel's masking results that have probably led to blindsight patients not having been tested on semantically rich material, and the question of the degree of similarity between the two domains—blindsight and backward masking—must await more systematic direct comparisons, extending the work along this line that Marcel himself has initiated.

There are two additional features of Marcel's findings of some relevance to issues concerning residual function. The first is that the attitude of the subject appears to be crucial, which will lead us in due course to the question of response criteria. The second is the question of whether or not it can be inferred which level of the nervous system might be involved, which will also be dealt with in a separate section below. As regards the subject's attitude, it will be noted in Fig. 32 that in the right hand panel all the functions are collapsed on to each other (and are approximately the same as the presence/absence function in the left hand panel). These were the results for subjects who were not passive: 'they felt the task to be nonsensical once they could not be sure of whether a stimulus was present, but had continued with the similarity judgments by adopting some idiosyncratic strategy'. These subjects Marcel called the 'strategy' subjects. The 'passive' subjects, on the other hand, whose results are shown in the left panel of the figure, 'mostly reported that they had at first been uncomfortable in judging similarity when they had to guess presence or absence, but had adopted a "passive" attitude and chosen the word which "felt" right'. (1983a, p. 204).

In testing a variety of subjects with visual field defects in which they are asked to 'guess' about a stimulus they cannot 'see', this feature of the problem is bound to strike any investigator. There are some subjects with whom testing simply has to be abandoned because they refuse to 'play the guessing game'. Perenin, Ruel, and Hécaen (1980, p. 608) remark of their patient with residual function that the forced-choice procedure was used 'irrespective of the patient's conscious visual experience, i.e., even if he did not really see anything'. They add somewhat wryly, 'Of course, he often took some time to be persuaded to do so'. In extreme cases, we have had subjects who resolutely say that they will not 'lie' by choosing such and such a stimulus when they 'know' that they can see that there is nothing there! No doubt the attitude of the investigator can also play an important role in this regard. If the subject is pressed to attend to the fine nuances of any weak visual stimulus, to be a 'conscientious' subject, he may fail, and this could be the explanation of failures to find 'blindsight' in some subjects and in some laboratories, or to find benefits of retraining. D.B.'s comment that he did not tire when doing forced-choice judgements in his blind field is especially apposite: 'I am not tired; I haven't been doing anything'. The disruptive effect of those stimuli in parts of the field that generated 'waves' has also been commented upon (see Chapter 13).

(d) Response criteria

The question of the subject's attitude raises in a direct way the formal issue of criterion levels. Perhaps subjects are more ready to acknowledge that a stimulus has been detected or is above threshold along a particular dimension in some modes of testing than in others. Or perhaps certain kinds of instructions induce different response criteria for different kinds of stimuli, 'degraded' in contrast to 'undegraded'. In terms that are equivalent, perhaps subjects are more willing to take risks under some stimulus conditions or some psychophysical procedures than under others. Signal detection theory was designed to analyse such a factor independently of discriminability *per se*.

It might seem, as all of the procedures involved in testing residual function are examples of psychophysical determinations, that if these two factors, discriminability (d') and response criterion (β) could be measured and contrasted for the intact and the defective fields, the issues in blindsight would be fully described and wholly resolved. The attraction to do so is seductive, and a few have succumbed easily to the charms. This is not to say that the values would not be without interest, but they do not provide an exhaustive or incisive answer to the particular problems of blindsight research. On the contrary, on closer examination they indicate what remains to be explained.

There are a number of ways in which it might be thought that an analysis of response criteria could be helpful. The first is to contrast the implicit psychophysical methods involved in perimetry, which produce a diagnosis of 'blindness', and the forced-choice methods used in blindsight, which yield evidence of good residual sensitivity. It might be hypothesized that the making of the response, 'now I see it' in perimetry yields a very conservative criterion, whereas forced-choice methods may allow a more lax attitude. But a change in response criterion *per se* cannot yield a change in sensitivity (d'). It is highly mischievous, one might venture, for Campion *et al.* to suggest that 'shift to a more lax criterion [with forced-choice response in the field defect] . . . restores performance (measured by the number of hits) to the sighted field level'. (1983, p. 427). Of course, the number of hits will increase with a relaxation of criterion, but so will the number of false alarms, and there can be no gain in sensitivity as such. In more technical language, the ROC curve is a curve of 'isosensitivity', to use Luce's term, and while some points on it may yield a better 'pay-off' than others according to the schedule of differential rewards and punishments for hits and false alarms, that is an entirely separate matter (cf. Lee 1971) from the one that is relevant here. A change in response criteria cannot affect sensitivity as such.

As it happens, forced-choice responding does characteristically yield a somewhat higher level of sensitivity (d′) than yes/no responding, but that is because the subject is given two presentations rather than one on which to make his judgements (Lee 1971). But in our experience the effect with D.B. was not large. The advantage in our situation (see Chapter 6) of thresholds determined by forced-choice responding over 'method of limits' (which Campion *et al.* also, with no strong justification, say will 'enforce a conservative criterion', 1983, p. 432, akin to that of perimetry) was seen to be rather small—of the order of 0.3 to 0.47 of a log unit.

In fact, there is no strong evidence that D.B.'s response criteria (or those of any other blindsight patient) in using forced-choice guesses were unduly lax. As it happens, most of the determinations yielded false positive rates too low to make ROC plotting profitable. But even when D.B. was approximately at threshold in 'presence vs. absence' (78%), his false-positive rate was only 18 per cent. Stoerig *et al.* (1985) deliberately set out to vary β in a blindsight patient and succeeded in doing so over a range from strict to lax, by adjusting the proportion of stimuli to blanks. The patient's capacity to detect stimuli in the scotoma remained more or less impervious to such variations in criterion level.

Slight shifts in sensitivity or even large variations in response criteria associated with different psychophysical procedures entirely miss the heart of the problem. This can be made clear by considering the difference between the 'blind' and the intact fields in D.B. when the *same* forced-choice methods are used in both. For example, we can measure detection by forced-choice methods in the blind field, as we have done for D.B. We can measure detection in precisely the same way in the intact field. We can define thresholds in terms of number of hits relative to false alarms, or in any other quantitatively consistent way. For each field we arrive at a threshold, calculated, say, as the 80 per cent correct response. (Whether or not the two fields have a different threshold in terms of physical energy or other parameters is, at this stage, irrelevant, because by definition performances at threshold are matched.) The point is that D.B. still resolutely refuses to agree that two stimuli equally above threshold (in terms of standard error units, if the purist insists) *are* equivalent, because one he says he sees, and the other he says he does not. An approach from signal detection theory simply fails to capture this difference. Werth (1983) has pointed out this fundamental difficulty succinctly. And, indeed, despite the wide range of response criteria imposed on their subject by Stoerig *et al.* (above), 'over and over again he claimed that he had no sensation whatsoever, that he was only guessing, and could hardly believe that his performance was above chance'. Werth (1983, p. 467) makes the same point: 'a patient's unawareness of visual stimuli may remain if a forced-choice procedure is applied, regardless of the response criterion the patient adopts'.

Nor should it be assumed that D.B. switched into a different mode or response state when doing forced-choice guessing that applied to all visual discriminations across the whole visual field. If even a slight amount of light happened to slip into the good field when we were working near the vertical meridian, or the apparatus happened to be misaligned (on one occasion, for example, the calibration on the control dial of the Aimark perimeter slipped by 7°), he was very quick to tell us. He was punctilious about reporting 'seen' events while he was, at the same time, tuned into 'guessing' about 'unseen' events.

In one way, intuitively it would appear that a more promising approach from signal detection theory would concentrate on d' rather than β. Given that typically D.B. (and other similar subjects) have raised thresholds for many types of visual discrimination in their field defect, as determined by forced-choice judgements of 'unseen' stimuli, it might be thought that actually to 'see', in the proper sense, requires a stimulus far above threshold, and not lying in the shadowy, marginal region near threshold. Perhaps D.B. perforce is confined to that somewhat unsatisfactory and murky zone separating signal from noise. That would be true in normal vision, as well: at near threshold values, as is well known, performance may be above chance even though the subject himself is uncertain. But normal subjects would typically say that they confidently actually 'see' when they are performing perfectly or near-perfectly at the 95–100 per cent level in a forced-choice discrimination task. But not D.B. As we have seen in several examples (e.g., movement, acuity, and orientation discriminations) he could consistently score at such levels and yet fail to acknowledge any experience. And so, just as the particular value of β is irrelevant, an explanation in terms of an inability to achieve a d' of high sensitivity using forced-choice guesses will not do either.

Of course, given that a blindsight subject 'sees' the stimulus in his good field, and is required to 'guess' the value of an unseen stimulus in his impaired field, it would not be surprising if the response criteria for the two psychophysical functions *were* different. It would be surprising, perhaps, if they were not. But whether one is more likely to be more lax than the other cannot be assumed *a priori*; it will no doubt depend on the subject, the instructions, and probably the stimulus dimension itself and, as we have seen, it can be made to vary over a wide range (Stoerig *et al.*) with complete irrelevance to the main problem. But the point is that it is parsimonious to assume that any difference in response criteria stems from the different modes of processing employed in the two fields, not vice versa. From this point of view, for example, that the slopes of the psychophysical functions for minimal separable acuity may appear to be different between D.B.'s impaired and intact fields is essentially trivial. (Nor, on a purely technical point, can it be assumed that the relatively poorer threshold for the amblyopic crescent stems purely from having used a different psychophysical method, done as a matter of convenience. Campion *et al.* (1983) appear incorrectly to argue that the threshold value would have been markedly different—more than an order of magnitude—if determined by forced-choice methods as was used for the blind field.)

But, again following an intuitive line of argument, one might say, if a signal detection analysis of the forced-choice guessing discrimination itself is not adequate, this may be because there are really *two* forced-choice judgements involved in the blindsight subject's performance. One is the forced-choice guessing discrimination itself under scrutiny, such as horizontal grating vs. non-horizontal grating but there is also an implicit 'seeing' vs. 'not seeing' choice to be made. Perhaps for the latter we need a really very large stimulus difference for a blindsight subject. But rather than providing an explanation, that is precisely the phenomenon that requires an explanation. One could with formal purity, ask D.B. to make a forced-choice response after each trial: 'see?' or 'not see?' He would resolutely say 'not see' on each occasion. His level of confidence is high that he does not see. Admittedly, with some dimensions and some situations, if the stimulus intensity were made very powerful, or if movement made very vigorous, he might then admit that he 'felt' or 'saw'. But the point is that the difference in sensitivity for forced-choice guessing and for forced-choice 'seeing' is very much larger, and may even be infinite, for the 'blind' field, in relation to such a difference in the intact field. That is the nub of the problem, and an analysis in terms of response criteria would at best provide mere descriptors but not explanations. The powerful hammer of signal detection theory may hit a nail, but it is not the one that requires driving here.

(e) Neural levels and pathways

To the extent that the properties of blindsight are the same as those used in responding to stimuli 'degraded' by visual masking (an identity not established) it would seem intuitively reasonable to argue that neither requires the use of a different neural route than is used for undegraded stimulus processing. But, in fact, visual masking could well involve a switch of pathways and of levels. Marcel found, for example, that his results were obtained only with 'central' backward masking, not with 'peripheral' masking. Central masking is obtained only with a contoured masking pattern, can only be obtained with backward (not forward) masking, and works both monoptically and dichoptically. Peripheral masking is directly affected by the energy of the masking field, and works with a blank or noise masking field, and works only monoptically (cf. Marcel 1983b; Turvey 1973). In other words, peripheral masking is most reasonably assumed to affect signal strength at a retinal or pregeniculate level, and central masking at a postgeniculate level, when there is binocular integration and interaction. If a central masking stimulus effectively destroys the strength of signal at the first cortical stage, area 17, other sub-cortical pathways may still be left open and receive their usual undegraded inputs. Further lexical processing might, then, occur at a more anterior cortical locus to which the sub-cortical signal might be relayed via the pulvinar. All this is, of course, speculation but is engaged in here merely to show that there is more than one possible explanation of neural pathways involved in the processing of centrally masked stimuli and that striate cortex could conceivably be bypassed. Not altogether fancifully, that is, central masking might be equivalent to striate cortex inactivation. What could be very interesting as a critical test, would be to see whether central masking in the scotoma destroyed the ability of a blindsight patient to process information with forced-choice guessing. If central masking effectively inactivates striate cortex, it should leave the capacity of the patient unaffected if striate cortex has already been destroyed. On the other hand, if the blindsight patient is still using striate cortex that has become relatively but not absolutely dysfunctional, central masking should be effective.

Be that as it may, as the formal similarity between blindsight and central masking is by no means established, one must consider the question of neural pathways that allows residual function in D.B.'s field defect to be effected, based upon the direct evidence of his test results and his verbal reports. It must be said, at once, that we do not know the precise details of his lesion — nor that of any other blindsight case. Both CT scan and NMR imaging are not useful or possible in D.B.'s case, given that the surgeons used metal clips to close his wound, and in any event their resolution is unlikely to be adequate. The surgical notes are, of course, very useful as a guide, but they too cannot give absolutely precise limits of extent or depth. That *some* striate cortex has been damaged seems a very safe assumption, but beyond that one must try to consider the various alternative possibilities.

The most conservative possibility is that there is not a problem to be considered — that striate cortex has not been completely damaged or destroyed, and wherever residual function can be found in the impaired field — whether or not he can report it — there must be at least partially functioning striate cortex. Whether or not verbal report would be exhibited would depend on response criteria and the relative severity of the dysfunction (or an artefact due to stray light). But unless one wishes to argue that there is, indeed, a discontinuity between monkey and man, and moreover that in none of the cases — including the hemidecortication patients of Perenin and Jeannerod, and several others that allow reasonable and conservatively based inferences about destruction of tissue from surgical or imaging information — was there an absolute destruction of striate cortex, this possibility seems far too unlikely. We have addressed the issues of artefact and response criteria and, if one assumes that striate cortex (or the input via the radiations) has been destroyed in some cases, then there is a genuine problem to be discussed. To dismiss it is more radical than to address it.

One possibility would be that the 'dead' part of the field, where D.B. reports no experience but can nevertheless make orientation and other discriminations, corresponds to a region for which the striate cortical projection has been completely destroyed. Those regions which are 'lively', but not veridical ('waves', 'jaggedness', 'something coming out', etc.) might correspond to partially but not completely destroyed striate cortex, and the intact part of the half-field, including the portion that recovered in 1976 when the scotoma shrank, to entirely intact striate cortex. The previously defective, but now recovered portion, may have had diminished blood supply which, for some reason, was restored. It is even possible that 'training' can act by increasing blood supply to striate cortex surrounding the absolute lesion, or alternatively, as suggested for the monkey, that lateral overlap in the projection to striate cortex might be exploited. Where there has been a qualitative recovery of normal function, i.e., colour, acuity, shape, and acknowledged report of veridical perception, as in the areas of recovered field in Zihl and von Cramon's cases, and the recovered portion of the upper field of D.B., it seems reasonable to assume that intact striate cortex has come into play.

But for those portions that remain relatively impaired, there is a more extreme possibility, namely that *all* the residual function (including 'waves', 'feeling', etc.) is subserved entirely by non-striate pathways — either in the midbrain or in the prestriate cortex (see Chapter 1). Those features of D.B.'s 'blind' vision — movement, orientation, localization, and reduced but preserved acuity — are precisely the discriminative capacities that have been demonstrated in monkeys with confirmed destruction of striate cortex, and moreover, as far as one can judge, they are quantitatively of the same order of magnitude. Mohler and Wurtz (1977) have shown very clearly that a midbrain pathway is critically involved in mediating the residual capacity for detection and localization within the field defect caused by a striate cortex lesion in the monkey. It is also the case that the residual capacity of the monkey diminishes as the lesion expands to include more extra-striate tissue in addition to striate cortex.

There is an even more extreme possibility which turns on the question of the age of the subject when the brain damage originally occurred. With D.B., it is quite possible that the angioma was present from birth, or at least from an early age. With the hemidecorticated patients of Perenin and Jeannerod there was also a suggestion that the degree of residual function correlated negatively with the age of the original brain damage. Damasio *et al.* (1975) report a striking case of a 34-year-old woman who had brain damage at the age of five, and a left hemispherectomy at the age of 20. Immediately after surgery the fields were markedly constricted (and the left eye virtually blind because of optic atrophy), but with the right eye 14 years later 'on the right she has almost normal vision. Testing of visual fields showed *no hemianopia*. Moreover, the field was enlarged as compared with the chart 14 years previously. The lack of hemianopia and the enlargement of the field were confirmed with repeated and spaced observations by different examiners'. (p. 90). Given that only the right eye could be used, there is a possibility, perhaps that the subject was using eccentric fixation, but given that it would be necessary for this to be quite marked (30°–40°), and given that the eyes were apparently under direct observation (for eye movements) in a perimeter when testing for slowly moving targets, this seems an unlikely possibility, although direct confirmation by plotting of the position of the optic disc would have been useful.

A truly remarkable case is reported by Jelsma in the discussion that follows Marquis's classical paper on encephalization of function (1935). It concerns a boy with a porencephalic cyst, presumably of prenatal origin, in the posterior left hemisphere, which was removed surgically at the age of 11 years. Jelsma states, 'we are certain as to the absence of the occipital lobe'. (p. 813). The boy's vision was remarkable. There was only slight constriction on the right, and normal zonal sensitivity to colour. Marquis himself saw the boy and was also present at surgery and made measurements of normal brains for comparison. In the ensuing discussion, he confirms Jelsma's observations, and agrees 'the entire occipital lobe, with the complete calcarine fissure, was lacking'. (p. 815). The confirmation is especially noteworthy given Marquis's clear endorsement, in the parent article, of the view that destruction of the calcarine cortex in humans normally leads to total and absolute blindness.

That field defects *do* occur in children with occipital damage is commonly reported, but their areal extent and functional density, in relation to the size of lesion and age of which it occurred, are not known. It is even possible that hemispherectomy might put sufficient demand on midbrain structures such that their maximal potential capacity could be exploited more readily than with smaller lesions at an early age. But for older subjects a more parsimonious view would seem reasonable that the integrity of posterior non-striate cortex is necessary. Clearly, studies of field defects caused by striate cortex lesions that occur early in life, and especially with long survival times, would be of considerable practical and theoretical interest.

But on the assumption that in subjects like D.B. extra-striate pathways might fully account for the residual capacity in the field defect, what then would be the neural basis for the distinction between residual capacity of which D.B. is 'aware', and for that of which he is not? The monkey evidence cannot, by itself, answer such a question, at least not in its present state. There would seem to be, in principle, two main possibilities, given that we accept the question as meaningful. The first is that there may only be a quantitative difference: that as stimuli become increasingly 'salient', they are increasingly likely to reach a strength above which the 'commentary system' (see below) is reliably activated. By 'salient' one would mean those stimulus properties constrained by the specific receptor sensitivities of the non-striate system. As more and more of the non-striate system were to become damaged, so more and more salience would be required for awareness to occur. The second possibility is that there is, indeed, a qualitative distinction between vision with 'awareness' and vision without, and that this reflects a different neural organization for each. It may be, of course, that increasing 'salience' of a stimulus will make it more likely to effect a switch to a different system, and so that is not a difficulty in itself. It seems likely that such a system would itself be cortical and, in man, involve a verbal capacity. Midbrain receptive areas project, via the thalamus, to the posterior non-striate cortex, and it might be that particular regions or combinations of regions of such cortex must be activated to enable us to say that we are 'aware' of a visual event. This is a possibility that is interesting to pursue, because it raises more general questions about the organization of a system said to mediate 'awareness', not only for vision but for other modalities and other systems (e.g., memory), but we defer discussion of these topics to a later section. First it is useful to review another approach, empirically based, to the question of the neural level involved in blindsight. How good is the correspondence between the properties of residual vision and the functional properties of *non-striate pathways*, as assessed in physiological and anatomical studies?

(f) Differential physiological and anatomical properties of striate vs. non-striate pathways

All of the relevant evidence is necessarily derived from animal research, and it also must be regarded as incomplete. Moreover, one cannot infer from the properties near the input stage what further transformations might occur before the output stage. To take a familiar example, cells in the dorsal lateral geniculate nucleus are not sensitive to the orientation of a signal on the retina. Exquisite orientation selectivity is first seen at the very next way-station, the striate cortex, and therefore must reflect the way in which lateral geniculate outputs converge upon striate cortex cells. Therefore, because recordings in the superior colliculus are not orientation selective does not preclude such a selectivity arising at a later stage from convergence upon cells upon which they project. On the other hand, one can confidently rule out the possibility that any later stage could itself introduce a sensitivity outside the band width at the earlier stage. If, to take a hypothetical example, receptors feeding into the non-striate pathway could not respond to a signal of less than such-and-such a level of light intensity, no further sensitivity to lower intensity signals could be generated later in the system. Therefore the most useful information about the constraints upon properties of non-striate pathways stems from the limits imposed at input. But even this cannot be a final determination, because the later projections from non-striate pathways may interact with the outputs from intact striate cortex (unless, rarely in the clinical literature, there is complete destruction of striate cortex *bilaterally*, which makes such cases especially useful). For example, a non-striate output may 'prime' cells specialized for colour perception, for which only the striate pathways appear to be specialized at an early stage.

Information about the anatomical and physiological sensitivities of striate vs. non-striate pathways in the primate is far from complete, but there is strong evidence that they are functionally distinct at an early stage. The evidence has been succinctly reviewed by Cowey (1985), and can be summarized briefly here. Ganglion cells of the retina, the axons of which constitute the optic nerve, are of four types, P-α, P-β, P-γ, and P-ϵ. (The 'P' refers to 'primate'.) Of these, the great majority are P-β, which have a projection exclusively to the striate cortex via the parvocellular layers of the dorsal lateral geniculate nucleus, and moreover *only* beta cells project to those layers of the lateral geniculate nucleus (cf. Perry *et al.* 1984). P-β cells are small and have relatively small dendritic fields. Physiologically they are 'colour'-opponent (strictly speaking, spectrally opponent), have slow conduction velocities, small receptive fields, and are 'X-like' in showing linear spatial summation within the receptive field. These cells, with information destined exclusively for striate cortex, clearly qualify as the substrate of a colour-opponent system with high-resolving power. Moreover, they form about 85 per cent of the ganglion cells in the fovea region of the eye.

The midbrain region receives inputs, in contrast, from predominantly P-γ and P-ϵ cells (Perry and Cowey 1984). Both are similar in having large and sparsely branched dendritic trees. They constitute about 10 per cent of the ganglion cells of the retina, giving rise to about 110 000 optic nerve fibres. Their properties can be studied by first identifying them by antidromic stimulation of their terminals in the superior colliculus (De Monasterio 1978; Schiller and Malpeli 1977). They have large receptive fields, poorly defined spatial opponency, non-linear spatial summation, low conduction velocities, and no colour opponency. They cannot be easily grouped in 'transient' or 'sustained'. A small proportion of P-α cells also project to the midbrain, but the large majority of P-α cells project to striate cortex via the dorsal lateral geniculate nucleus. (Interestingly, however, that projection to striate cortex is segregated from the P-β cell projection. P-α cells project via different layers of the geniculate, the magnocellular, and their termination in striate cortex has a different laminar disposition, in fine detail, than the P-β cells projecting via the parvocellular layers of the geniculate.)

The recently discovered direct projection from the monkey geniculate to pre-striate cortex (see Chapter 1) appears to comprise about one per cent or less of the lateral geniculate neurons. They are distributed throughout all layers of the geniculate, and are intermediate in size between parvo- and magnocellular neurones of the geniculate. Nothing is known of their physiological properties. Of the remaining projections to destinations other than midbrain and pre-striate cortex, such as hypothalamus, ventral lateral geniculate, accessory optic tract nucleus, nothing is known of the character of the anatomical classification of ganglion cells of origin or the physiological properties of these small pathways.

There is a remarkable phenomenon that allows conclusions to be drawn directly about the classes of retinal ganglion cells involved in residual vision after striate cortex damage. After striate cortex ablation, both in man and in monkey, many of the ganglion cells of the retina degenerate (van Buren 1963; Cowey 1974). This process must obviously be trans-neuronal, as the ganglion cells do not project directly to the striate cortex (but indirectly via a relay in the lateral geniculate). It was originally thought that the degeneration affected mainly the ganglion cells in the macular region, resulting in a more or less uniform density of cells across the whole retina similar to that of the normal peripheral retina (Cowey 1974). More recently it appears that the density gradient is not flat, but shows the normal decrease in the numbers of cells from central to peripheral retina (Cowey and Perry, personal communication; for discussion of the technical problems involved cf. Perry *et al.* 1984). Thus, there is an approximately normal density gradient, but much reduced in absolute level.

By placing a retrograde labelling substance (horseradish peroxidase) into the optic nerve after transneuronal degeneration has taken place, it has proved possible to identify the types of ganglion cells that remain intact in the retina (Cowey and Perry 1985). Not surprisingly, the majority of P-β cells have degenerated. Many P-α cells remain intact, although most must project to the 'missing' magnocellular portion of the lateral geniculate. However, the P-γ and P-ϵ cells are intact, and therefore one can conclude that the residual visual capacity in monkey, and presumably in man, are mediated by these P-γ and P-ϵ cells, together with a small number of P-α cells. As the electrophysiological properties of these cell types have been studied, it is possible to relate them to the spectrum of residual capacities after striate cortex lesions.

Several workers have drawn parallels between the properties of the residual vision both in destriate monkeys and of human patients, on the one hand, and the properties of the midbrain pathways, on the other. We have seen that the latter are anatomically segregated from the striate system, even at the stage of initial input from the retinal ganglion cells, and show qualitatively distinct physiological response characteristics, strongly suggesting a functionally dissociable role. There is a topological map of the visual field in the colliculus, which could allow spatial localization to occur. The relationship between collicular single unit activity and saccadic eye movements, especially the 'enhancement' effect, provides a link both with eye movement localization in blindsight studied by many workers since Pöppel *et al.*'s first study (1973), as well as the attentional phenomena studied by Singer *et al.* (1977). Units in the colliculus of monkey are selectively sensitive to flashed and moving stimuli (Schiller and Koerner 1971; Goldberg and Wurtz 1972), and there is reasonable correspondence between psychophysical data on sensitivity with target velocity in Patient G. (Barbur *et al.* 1980). The colliculus of monkey receives an input, albeit a small one, from the P-α cells of the retina, which are fast conducting, have large receptive fields, are highly contrast sensitive, and are often considered to have a specialized role for detection of transient visual signals. The large spatial summation area shown by Patient G. is also in line with the large receptive fields of P—γ, P-ϵ and P-α cells, which would also be in accord with the reduced visual acuity of D.B. The lack of spectral selectivity of collicular units would also be in agreement with all the clinical findings. Some of the clinical findings, e.g., the low critical fusion frequency of G., suggest what further properties of P-γ and P-ϵ cells in the retina, and single units in the colliculus, might be investigated electrophysiologically.

In general, it can be said that there is reasonable correspondence between the response properties of the non-striate receptors and pathways, and the capacities of residual visual function in patients with field defects caused by lesions of the striate cortex. While the correspondences are not sufficiently complete empirically, and are not of a precision to rule out other alternative explanations of residual function (e.g., 'patchy' islands of relatively dysfunctional striate cortex), heuristically there is little doubt that the characterization of the non-striate system as a qualitatively distinct partner within the framework of the 'two visual system' hypothesis has been very productive in furthering and organizing thinking about clinical phenomena and blindsight. This general hypothesis stemmed from animal research (see Chapter 1) that suggested that striate cortex lesions interfered with the identification of visually presented objects, but not with their detection and localization. Conversely, collicular lesions in animals cause impaired orienting responses towards visual stimuli and a reduction in responses to novel targets (Schneider 1967; Goodale and Lister 1974; Goodale and Murison 1975; Goodale, Foreman, and Milner 1978; Milner, Goodale, and Morton 1979; Milner, Lines, and Migdal 1984; Heywood and Cowey 1985). It is also of interest that patients with midbrain pathology show reduced latency of orienting responses (cf. Posner, Cohen, and Rafal 1982; Goodale 1980; Heywood and Ratcliff 1976). William James put it very well in a slightly different connection: 'The main function of the peripheral part of the retina is that of sentinels which, when beams of light move over them, cry: "Who goes there?" and calls the fovea to the spot' (1892, p. 73). It is no accident that the 'second visual system' has also been linked with ambient vision (Trevarthen 1968), but the James quote is readily converted into two-visual system thinking by substituting 'mid-brain' for 'peripheral part of the retina', and 'striate cortex' for 'fovea'.

The spectrum of D.B.'s residual function also fits in well with the general framework of a qualitatively different system, based on different cells of origin and different terminals, and with a different function. He can detect and locate, but has difficulty in identifying either in the sense of making forced-choice responses between shapes that do not have good local orientation cues, or in the obvious sense that his choices can be devoid of any acknowledged awareness. Acuity and other psychophysical functions decline with increasing eccentricity, in line with the falling density gradient of P-ϵ and P-γ cells. The bias towards experiencing transient stimuli might depend upon the intact P-α ganglion cells. Nevertheless, his ability to respond to sustained stimuli (see Chapter 9) could be mediated by non-transient midbrain cells. There is a discrepancy between his good ability to discriminate orientation in the frontal plane and the insensitivity of collicular single units to the orientation of retinal stimuli. However, just as with the transform from the 'orientation-less' units of the lateral geniculate nucleus to those of the striate cortex with their exquisite sensitivity to orientation, so there may be a transform beyond the colliculus that would allow orientation to be selectively processed. In any event, it is noteworthy, in this connection, that the monkey with confirmed total striate cortex removal can discriminate orientation differences of about 8°, and hence non-striate pathways *are* patently capable of mediating such a discrimination at some stage. If D.B. and similar patients turn out to have the lexical decision capacities of Marcel's patients, then the later stages of processing, no doubt via relays to posterior cortical regions, have a much greater burden to carry, but that possibility awaits further research.

(g) 'Awareness' and the definition of 'blindsight'

The complete positivistic sceptic can leave us at this stage. 'From the theoretical point of view the unconscious aspect of blindsight is hence [because of signal detection response criteria as an alternative description] essentially trivial, and from the practical point of view it is impossible to treat scientifically'. (Campion *et al.* 1983, p. 427). But the problem that has captured the interest of blindsight researchers did not emerge from a mysterious vapourous mist, but directly from the study of the patients themselves and in their relation to behavioural and physiological evidence from animals. It was the disjunction between their verbal reports and their discriminative capacity that was surprising. The question now is what status (in 'scientific' terms) to attach to these verbal reports?

In strict behaviourist tradition, one could simply treat verbal reports as behavioural responses, empty of any experiential or 'non-scientific' content. Note that in strictly formal terms there is just as much rigour in treating the choice between conscious 'seeing' vs. 'not seeing' as there is between 'guessing x' vs. 'guessing non-x' without 'awareness'. In both cases the psychophysical procedure is identical; it is only the response categories that differ. The only validation that ever occurs in psychophysics derives from the correspondence between controlled variations along a stimulus dimension and the probability of a response. Therefore in postulating two psychophysical functions, one for 'seeing' and the other for 'guessing' (see above, Section (d)), there is no more mystery about one than the other, and neither is less 'trivial' in operational terms. The validation for both psychophysical functions entails precisely the same operations, even though to the subject the response categories are markedly different in meaning.

But even at the operational level, there is a *practical* aspect in the context of blindsight that derives from the disjunction between verbal reports of 'seeing' and forced-choice 'guessing'. Verbal responses, in response to verbal questions by the examiner, are the bread and butter of the clinical assessment of sensory capacity, and one of the points to emerge clearly from blindsight research is that they may seriously underestimate residual capacity. The present topic has arisen, after all, because researchers normally are content to listen trustingly to the subjects' verbal reports. The forced-choice methods, deriving from animal research, may uncover much more than verbal methods, and retraining methods may allow such a capacity to be developed further even if the patient himself has no awareness of the capacity. But, of course, the converse is also true: verbal reports can reveal more than non-verbal reports, and the reason is that the examiner, like all of us in our daily interactions, assumes that the verbal response *does* have content and reference. This is one reason why we learn something from testing the sensory capacities of human subjects that is virtually impossible from testing animals, at least without a very great deal more time, if ever. We shall assume here that such a verbal reference is usually to phenomenal experience (only 'usually', because verbal reports can themselves be automatic and devoid of any corresponding experience as a referent.)

The reasons for making straight away what may seem to some to be such a bold jump (although the average man treats the existence of phenomenal experience in himself and others as mundane and self-evident) are several: first, there seems to be no other easy way in terms of a universal human discourse to capture the difference between the reports of subjects' responses to supra-threshold stimuli in the 'blind' vs. the 'seeing' fields. We have already reviewed the stiuation that arises with such stimuli when thresholds are measured in the two fields by precisely the same psychophysical methods. With supra-threshold stimuli for orientation, movement, or detection, we may find a virtually perfect performance, and yet the subject is adamant that they are quite different in quality: he is patently aware of one but not the other. If pressed, he does not say, 'I can make a verbal response to one but not the other'; he insists that they give rise to different experiences.

A second reason stems from other advances in neurology that have come from a direct acceptance of the level of phenomenal report. As Underwood has put it, 'if we are not to ask humans about their beliefs about their internal states, then a great deal of activity in psychology and medicine is called into question'. (1983, p. 463). It is doubtful whether anaesthetics would have been produced or trusted if subjects' reports of their experiences (or their memories of them) were not assumed to have some reality. If a dentist were trying out a new local anaesthetic on us before drilling into the nerve or pulling a tooth, he had better assume that our experience has some reality! But one can go beyond this and cite examples where our understanding of neural events themselves could not have advanced without reports of phenomenal experience. A nice example is of the correlation between REM (rapid eye-movement) sleep and dreams. That relationship could not have been discovered if one did not wake human subjects during different EEG phases of sleep, and ask about their experiences. REM sleep would have remained, in principle, forever incomprehensible without an appeal, at some stage, to some aspect of reports of experience. If a phenomenal report can advance neurology in such a mode, why not in the analysis of visual capacity? And, conversely, if phenomenal report can advance neurology, then neurology should also be able to advance our understanding of phenomenal report. Underwood has argued cogently that 'rather than to exclude [verbal reports] from any consideration, we must collect introspective reports as evidence. They are responses to sensory stimulation, and thus correspond to changes in the nervous system'. (1983, p. 464).

A third reason is a biological one: if it is universally accepted by ordinary men and women that we all have phenomenal experience, then what would be the evolutionary value of such a claim: not only for our belief in its existence, but even beyond to the reason for its very existence? The phenomenon of blindsight, and other 'non-conscious' processes, does at least challenge one to speculate about this and, in so doing, to put the matter in a biological and hence scientific context.

In allowing a legitimate status for phenomenal experience in our scientific discourse, it does not mean that philosophical questions regarding it are not tangled and complex, and we make no absurd claim here to find a ready answer to mind–body problems. Some philosophers, in fact, have found the evidence of 'blindsight' to have important philosophical implications (Searle 1979; Natsoulas 1982; Churchland 1980, 1983), but interesting as they are, they need not concern us directly, provided we can in principle work out scenarios involved in our everyday discourse when we try to relate our experiences to other persons' or to understand them. In the perceptual realm it no doubt has to do with a common assent growing out of ostensive procedures. We share our 'looking' and, usually, if we are looking together, our acknowledgement of 'seeing'. When someone reports 'seeing' something out of our own view, there is no difficulty in knowing the procedures for confirmation or convincing ourselves that he has a certain kind of experience. No doubt there are complex issues involved in trying to disentangle the status and meaning of hallucinations, or any experiences which cannot be shared — our 'private' experiences of our own bodies, our own pain, our own memories, etc. — but in principle their status can be understood in precisely the same way as shared experiences, except that there is no shared referent.

There is also the issue of the status of a verbal system as a concomitant, or even as a prerequisite for phenomenal experience and 'self-awareness'. Is there any way of determining whether animals, lacking a verbal system, have perceptual 'awareness'? This is a question to which we shall return, but it is not necessary, whatever epistemological and ontological questions may remain unsolved, for us to impose, as an act of ascetic self-denial, a prohibition on our considering how our nervous systems are organized to distinguish between those events of which we acknowledge 'awareness' and those that we process without 'awareness'. It is much easier, although it is still a very difficult challenge, to do this for a sensory mode where there is some common acceptance of what is meant universally by saying we are 'aware' of some visual event in the environment, than the more esoteric 'qualia' of raw feelings.

It is perhaps time to advance a definition of blindsight. No apology is needed for leaving it to such a late stage. Definitions are more helpful after one considers the body of background knowledge to a concept than before. In fact, the term crept into the field almost by stealth. I had to provide a title quickly for a local talk soon after the work with D.B. started, and concocted the title, with quadruple entendre, of 'Blindsight and hindsight'. The name stuck, and we used it in the title of a short article in the *Lancet* soon afterwards (Sanders *et al.* 1974), since when it is has been reified by many but rarely defined. As it seems likely that the name will be with us for some time, it may be better to try to define it than to eradicate it. The definition we suggest is: visual capacity in a field defect in the absence of acknowledged awareness. This leaves open the question of the pathways by which such capacity is mediated, although the animal work of course does suggest what the major candidates would be. Also the definition, as it stands, applies only to those subjects who can communicate to us whether or not they are aware. That implies a restriction to human subjects, but we do not think it meaningless to ask, and attempt to consider how an answer might be found, whether an animal also is aware of stimuli projected into its field defect. If there is to be a biological investigation of the question, one is more or less forced to think about it at the animal level.

(h) The commentary system

Thus far we have concentrated on what D.B. *can* do with stimuli within his field defect. We now turn to consider what he cannot do, and in particular the handicap that lack of awareness imposes on the processing of such stimuli. It is not yet clear from the evidence with D.B. or any of the other cases reviewed which of the two possibilities outlined above briefly (see above, Section (e)) best fits the relationship between stimuli of which he is aware and those of which he is not. To repeat, one possibility is that it may only be a quantitative difference based on 'salience' of stimulus events, as defined in terms of the triggering properties of the residual receptor system. The other is that there may be a different system involved in the two states, but that increasing salience may have an effect (among other factors) in bringing about a switch from one to the other. That salience *per se* is relevant comes from many observations with D.B. and pervades the accounts given earlier in the monograph. Depending on the location in the field, there is a standard progression starting from complete lack of awareness of stimulus events that he can discriminate, and resolute denial of any such awareness. With increasing stimulus salience, e.g., luminous contrast or velocity of movement, he may start to acknowledge a 'feeling' that something is happening and is usually able to locate where the feeling comes from in space. The feeling may have spatial properties, in the sense that he may feel that there is something coming out from the screen. It may also have a 'wave-like' impression, or be like 'moving my hand in front of my eyes when the room is totally dark'. He nevertheless denies that such feelings are 'seeing'. [The possible amodal quality of such a 'feeling' reminds one of Humphrey's observations with Helen, the monkey with striate cortex damage, who could detect and locate visual *or* auditory events in space, but had great difficulty in discriminating a visual from an auditory event, an extremely simple task for a normal monkey.] With still greater salience, D.B. may acknowledge genuine 'seeing', but this typically is not veridical. For example, with vigorous movement of a high contrast object, he may describe (and draw) what he sees as a curious set of distorted and bent lines.

A highly similar progression is seen in Barbur *et al.*'s patient, G. (Barbur, personal communication). Thus, with briefly flashed test stimuli having luminance values between 4 and 16 ft lamberts (against a background of 2.9 ft lamberts), G. 'categorically reports that he detects nothing at all and is not aware of anything'. But nevertheless Barbur and his colleagues find that the location of such targets exercise good control of saccadic eye movements. Above this level, e.g., a test target of about 41 ft lamberts, he lacks 'any kind of "perceived" component although he reports that he is somehow "aware" of something being presented in the blind hemifield'. At the highest retinal illuminance levels (available only in a Maxwellian system, up to 4 to 5 log trolands), 'G. reports a change in darkness level which he can localise in what he describes as "the emptiness" of his blind hemifield'.

But while stimulus strength, or salience, as determined by the sensitivity of the relevant receptors, is clearly an important variable in determining whether or not D.B. and other such subjects have acknowledged awareness, it does not follow that the contrasting states should be characterized simply as a quantitative progression along a dimension of strength of activation, as though 'becoming conscious of something is merely like opening a door to, or it being pushed by, one aspiring entrant'. (Marcel, 1983*b*, p. 250). On the contrary, it will be recalled that the 'waves', when they occurred, may well have interfered with D.B.'s performance, and he performed better on some tasks when the area was quite 'dead'. Also, a passive attitude, when there 'was nothing to do' because he 'did not see anything', may well facilitate performance for stimuli of which he is not conscious, just as it was said to do for Marcel's masking experiments and in the subception literature (Dixon 1971). Marcel reviews thoroughly the arguments, theoretical as well as empirical, for considering that a non-conscious process is not just a weaker copy of something that can be conscious, with otherwise similar processing rules. But whether the threshold for 'feeling' and the higher threshold for 'seeing' (non-veridical) is passed only along such a dimension of increasing salience, or whether 'seeing' requires other conditions as well and satisfies different requirements, a view to which we subscribe, is not relevant to the point immediately under consideration: namely, what value, in a biologically adaptive sense, attaches to being 'aware', and what is precluded by being 'unaware' (even though discriminative capacity can still be demonstrated)? What is the benefit, if any, of the door's opening, and the penalty for its remaining closed?

The biological value of conscious awareness is a topic that has not escaped a vast amount of discussion over the past century, and it would be rash to attempt to suggest a final outcome, even if one were possible. But the line of attack that seems relevant to this, and to some other neurological conditions, is one suggested by Lloyd Morgan almost 100 years ago. 'If a being has the power of thinking "thing" or "something", it has the power of transcending space and time. . . . Here is the point where intelligence ends and reason begins.' (Lloyd Morgan 1890, p. 375, quoting Mivart with approval). To be aware of a visual event is not only to be able to categorize it as a 'thing', i.e., to categorize it as a prototypical object independently of retinotopic space, but to have the capacity to treat that event as an image, to store it in that form, to match it or contrast it with other images, in short to think and to reflect 'visually'. A great deal of visual processing, even rather complex processing, can proceed automatically if it is based on discriminations that do not require reflection; all visuo-motor skills are of this character ultimately. On the assumption that there is a limited capacity for thought—that it is difficult to 'think about more than one thing at a time'—it would be wasteful in the extreme to occupy valuable cerebral capacity other than for thinking and imaging, unless one has the luxury of free time for idle thought and day-dreaming. A large amount of bodily processing, including in sensory channels, proceeds quite detached from any awareness. The pupillary response, for example, is continuously changing in response not only to luminance level in relation to adaptation level, but also to emotional and motivational states. No one is aware of the action of his pupil, nor is there any good reason that he should be, because its function can be executed quite automatically. Much more complex performances, like driving a car or playing tennis, similarly become automatic when they are practised and may even be seriously impeded if one tries to become aware of the fine components as the act progresses, a phenomenon that Stephen Potter exploited to full humorous effect in drawing up his list of 'gamesmanship' ploys. Awareness of an event is a form of privileged access that allows further perceptual and cognitive manipulations to occur; as far as neural processes are concerned, it is probably a minority privilege.

Being aware of an event not only goes with thinking but also, of course, with *communicating* with others. In fact, the question naturally arises whether somehow D.B. suffers from a syndrome of disconnection between the damaged visual cortex in the right hemisphere and the language areas of the left hemisphere, a result that could occur, for example, if the surgeons inadvertently (and improbably) cut the splenium of the corpus callosum. Perhaps, as is claimed for the commissurotomy ('split-brain') patients, D.B.'s lack of awareness arises from being unable to talk about his right hemisphere visual inputs. There are several reasons for rejecting this possibility. Firstly, if the splenium were cut it is unlikely that part of the left visual field would be preserved. Secondly, it does not matter whether D.B. uses a verbal or a non-verbal response to signal his discrimination. In the 'monkey' perimeter, he was required to indicate his 'guessing' of the location of a target with a verbal response ('near' vs. 'far'), unlike the typical Aimark perimeter situation, where he pointed silently with his hand. The issue is not whether the response is verbal or non-verbal, but the type of question that D.B. is attempting to answer, and the type of decision he attempts to make. The difference is between reacting and monitoring. Thirdly, over the blindsight field as a whole there are patients with left hemisphere visual cortex lesions, and these do not appear to behave any differently from those with right hemisphere lesions.

Finally, I was kindly given the opportunity by Professor Roger Sperry in 1975 to study two 'split-brain' patients in the California series (N.G. and A.A.), to see how close the similarity might be with D.B. The answer is that they were quite different. Indeed, when simple stimuli were presented tachistoscopically to their left half-visual fields of the type of which D.B. denied 'awareness', all of the patients discriminated correctly, and did so even with small stimuli, e.g., **X** vs. **O**, well below D.B.'s 'guessing' threshold, and could give reasonably accurate descriptions of their dimensions and locations on the screen. And, they insisted that they actually *saw* the stimuli, in just the same way as they could see them in their right half-fields; 'no trouble at all', said N.G. Other interesting observations of these two patients also emerged, but this is not the place to relate them. The point is that these two commissurotomy patients, frequently cited in the literature on that subject, appear to be qualitatively and quantitatively distinctly different from D.B.

It is not only in the area of blindsight that a disjunction between performance and acknowledged awareness occurs. We have already noted reports of a similar disjunction in some cases of prosopagnosia (Travel and

Damasio 1985) and 'blind touch' (Paillard *et al.* 1983). But even more striking examples, perhaps, and studied over a much longer period, are found in the area of memory disorders, in particular the amnesic syndrome, a neurological condition caused by damage to particular anatomical sites in the limbic lobe and diencephalon. Such severely incapacitated patients appear not to be able to remember events beyond a minute or two. We showed also (Warrington and Weiskrantz 1968) that they could, in fact, learn certain types of both verbal and pictorial material very well and could retain them over quite long periods. The evidence emerged from the use of techniques that do not require a subject to respond to a question about his *memory* for the material, but merely to give a response directly to a stimulus or cue which must depend for its successful elicitation upon the learning having occurred. But the amnesic patient does not acknowledge this or any other acquired information as a 'memory'.

This aspect of the amnesic syndrome was noted as long ago as 1911 by Claparède. MacCurdy placed considerable emphasis upon it as well in his 1928 book. There are now a number of different approaches to the theoretical implications, among them our own interpretation of the syndrome specifically in terms of a neural 'disconnexion syndrome' (Warrington and Weiskrantz 1982). Since 1968 the area has been one of considerable interest and activity, by no means free of debate (see Weiskrantz 1985a, for a review of some of the issues), but there is agreement among all workers in the field that there can be considerable and good retention of certain forms of material revealed by 'non-mnemonic' cues or by conditioning which the amnesic subject himself, however, resolutely fails to recognize or acknowledge as his own memory.

And so questions in our everyday lives that we find commonplace and mundane, such as 'what do you remember?', or 'can you recognize such and such?', or 'what do you see?' are rather more complex than they might appear. They are questions that refer not only to the result or outcome of a process, but also to a 'commentary' upon it. It is also commonplace that our 'commentaries' may be poor indicators of, or even elaborate constructions upon, the underlying processes, but phenomena such as blindsight demonstrate the preservation of a process in the total absence of acknowledged awareness where the two are normally closely linked, and moreover provide at least a starting point for considering the neural basis of such a disjunction.

What might that basis be? We have suggested that the commentary system is activated when we characteristically are able to carry out cognitive operations upon current or stored events, that is, to classify, to order, to rehearse, to imagine, to provide a 'schema' within which behaviour is initiated and directed, and to communicate. There are, from this viewpoint, several systems, as many as are found to be dissociable neuropsychologically (cf. Broadbent and Weiskrantz 1982). For visual events, the early input stages in the striate cortex, therefore, while they provide an entrée into such systems, would not be sufficient in themselves for acknowledged awareness. Stimulation of the striate cortex does give rise, in human subjects, to reports of scattered 'phosphenes', i.e., flashing lights, but it is of interest that in the monkey, removal of all *non*-visual cortex (but leaving motor cortex intact) is reported to render the animal clinically blind (Nakamura and Mishkin 1980). Thus, striate cortex *may* be necessary but it seems highly likely that it is not sufficient. Whether or not it is necessary is more difficult to decide. We can find no reports of stimulation of midbrain centres in awake human subjects to learn what kind of verbal reports are elicited (the output from the midbrain bypasses the striate cortex). Such observations would be of great interest, although the circumstances under which they could be ethically justified are very few. Perhaps the most parsimonious assumption is that with sufficiently strong activation of the midbrain, regions of cortex may be stimulated via thalamic relays from the midbrain, that partially activate regions of cortex involved in cognitive operations, but activate them only in a disorganized way that gives rise to non-veridical perception.

On the other hand, it was reported that with high contrast visual stimuli the unilateral neodecorticated human subjects of Perenin and colleagues are said to experience a 'feeling that a quite bright light had been turned on in the impaired part of their visual field, and was spreading from there into the normal field', although they did not 'see the form or size of the target, nor have any conscious idea about its location . . .' (Perenin 1978, p. 699). We have also noted the striking cases of apparently normal visual awareness in the absence of the calcarine cortex reported by Damasio *et al.* (1975) and by Jelsma (in Marquis 1935). And so it might be that not only is striate cortex unnecessary, but any neocortex at all is unnecessary! That is, under certain circumstances midbrain structures, without further relay to ipsilateral cortex, might be sufficient to mediate 'awareness'. This condition may depend, as noted above, on the occurrence of the lesion at an early age and, possibly, on the lesion being quite large and complete; usually a more parsimonious assumption would obtain.

Commentary type questions are probably the most common type of question we ask fellow humans. It is possible to ask them of animals? That is, to ask them not only what they can discriminate, which we can do routinely, but whether they *see*? In other words, is it possible that the monkey without striate cortex also has blindsight, is discriminating without awareness? Those who are uneasy or sceptical of such a question in relation to a human patient may well throw up their hands in despair when it is directed to the animal level. But if we accept a position of evolutionary continuity, there is no reason why we should not allow animals some 'awareness' in the same sense in which we have it, and therefore to allow that they also be made 'unaware' by the same type of neurological disconnection as in man. Darwin himself was convinced of the continuity, and commented, 'We have seen that the senses and intuitions, the various emotions and faculties, such as love, memory, attention, curiosity, imitation, reason, etc., of which man boasts, may be found in an incipient, or even sometimes in a well-developed condition, in the lower animals'. (1871, pp. 125–6).

The issue has been discussed elsewhere (Weiskrantz 1977, 1985b, in press), but briefly, it would appear necessary to pursue the matter experimentally, to separate the discrimination itself from a separate response category that would operate as a 'commentary' upon the discrimination. This was what has been done in an ingenious idea put forward by Beninger *et al.* (1974). In effect, they have asked laboratory rats if they know what they are doing. They allowed the rats to carry out any one of four possible acts (which were acts that rats do quite frequently and without training): (1) to face-wash, (2) to rear up, (3) to walk, or (4) to remain immobile. The animals could do any of these four acts in any order they wished. But in order to get food reward, after they performed any one of these acts they had to press one of four different response levers, so as to indicate what it was they had done. Rats can do this type of task. It would be very surprising if a monkey could not. It might also be surprising if a sea slug or crab *could* do it, but who knows?

More generally, one can provide a pair of keys for a forced-choice discrimination between two visual stimuli, and another pair for the 'commentary' alternatives. There are still a number of questions, both methodological and theoretical, that arise in such a task (among them, for example, the conversion to 'automatic' chaining of the two sets of responses with practice) which we cannot pursue here. But in principle it seems a possible approach. Certainly, D.B. would discriminate with one set of keys correctly between, say, two different orientations of a grating, but would respond with the 'do not see' commentary key (note that in the commentary set there is no 'correct' answer).

While the idea is reasonable in principle, it makes an interesting thought experiment to see how it might work in practice for a monkey. It would first have to be taught to operate the commentary keys. One would adopt the same methods as with a normal human subject (even a mute subject), namely to give examples of visual events which are clearly visible to us (and are known to be clearly discriminable to the subject), for which the 'see' commentary key would be appropriate, and others that are well below threshold (or do not occur at all), for which the 'do not see' key would be appropriate. At this stage the commentary keys would be differentially reinforced, in effect, for a distinctive 'presence' vs. 'absence' discrimination. Next, an independent discrimination would be established on the 'discrimination' keys, say, between gratings of two different orientations. The animal, at the next stage, would carry out both the 'discrimination' and the 'commentary' successively on each trial, but unlike the Beninger situation, without a contingency *between* the two phases.

The question is whether there would ever be a disjunction between the two sets of response alternatives as the discrimination became increasingly difficult, as with masking, or if the striate cortex were ablated, so that, for example, the orientation discrimination remained above chance even though the animal pressed the 'absence' key. Whether in practice such a regime could be established with a non-verbal creature is an open question, although the field of memory disorders mentioned above, where there is a similar separation between evidence of learning in the absence of acknowledged awareness of a 'memory', the task has, in effect, almost been completed. An animal with a lesion in the neural system known to be involved in the human amnesic syndrome will successfully learn and continue to perform a forced-choice visual discrimination between two objects. But in an independent test in the same apparatus (but not, as it happens, with the same stimuli), Gaffan (1974) has shown that the animals fail to *recognize* objects as familiar. The two phases could no doubt be put together and, just as with human amnesic patients, one would expect the animal to make a successful discrimination between stimuli he did not recognize as having seen before.

The experiment with 'discrimination' plus 'see/no see' would be a challenge in practice, especially if one could take it to the stage where the animal could successfully 'guess' the presence or absence of a stimulus event on the discrimination keys, even though he signalled 'not present' on a commentary key, as in effect is the case with D.B. The thought experiment itself is helpful in trying to work out in detail what the situation would require of a non-verbal creature (it might be easier with a chimpanzee who could be taught to sign 'see' vs. 'not see'). But at least in principle it would seem reasonable to approach the issue by separating 'commentary' responses from the discriminations themselves. Indeed, such a separation would seem to be an essential prerequisite for an enquiry into awareness, and hence into blindsight, to be approached at all. The advantage of such an approach is that, like the empirical findings that led to blindsight itself, it would allow the animal and human levels to share a common viewpoint.

As a concluding remark, I can confess that there was no idea, in advance, of how rich the outcome would be of studying this one person intensively and longitudinally. It was gratifying to see the similarity of the results with the animal findings, in objective terms, because it helps to bridge a gap that was becoming increasingly embarrassing and puzzling as animal work revealed more and more residual capacity in the absence of striate cortex. It had become clear that the non-striate pathways in animals were important bypasses. But the background of work on animals gave no hint that we would find such a striking dissociation between discriminative capacity and acknowledged awareness and hence that we would be required to delve into questions of the neurology of awareness. Quite aside from these theoretical and academic aspects, and the important dissociations that continue to emerge — especially, in the present context, between identification and orienting — it is also gratifying that the results, incomplete as they are, indicate unambiguously that the visual system damaged at the cortical level has a greater residual capacity for discrimination than is revealed by even quite searching clinical methods, or by the subject's own experience. Given the animal research, it is to be expected that there will also be greater capacity for recovery of function with training than had been appreciated. Just how this field of vision will shape up in the future is difficult to predict, but we are grateful to D.B.'s visual field, and to him personally, for helping us come this far. And, no matter what the precise limits of his cortical lesion happen to be (and we hope that it will be others, not us, who will learn that in the far distant future), we must thank him for making us think about the issues involved in the neuropsychology of visual perception.

References

Barbur, J. L., Ruddock, K. H., and Waterfield, V. A. (1980). Human visual responses in the absence of the geniculo-calcarine projection. *Brain* **102**, 905–28.

Bauer, R. M. and Rubens, A. B. (1985). Agnosia. In *Clinical neuropsychology* (eds. K. M. Heilman and E. Valenstein), pp. 187–241. Oxford Univ. Press, New York.

Bender, M. B. and Krieger, H. P. (1951). Visual function in perimetrically blind fields. *Arch. Neurol. Psychiat.* **65**, 72–9.

—— and Teuber, H-L. (1946). Phenomena of fluctuation, extinction and completion in visual perception. *Arch. Neurol. Psychiat.* **55**, 627–58.

Beninger, R. J., Kendall, S. B., and Vanderwolf, C. H. (1974). The ability of rats to discriminate their own behaviours. *Canad. J. Psychol.* **28**, 79–91.

Blythe, I. M., Kennard, C., and Ruddock, K. H. (1985). Residual function in hemianopia and quadrantanopia. Paper delivered at meeting of European Brain and Behaviour Society, Oxford.

Brain, W. R. (1981). *Brain's diseases of the nervous system.* (8th edn, revised by J. N. Walton.) Oxford University Press, Oxford.

Bridgeman, B. and Staggs, D. (1982). Plasticity in human blindsight. *Vision Res.* **22**, 1199–1203.

Brindley, G. S., Gautier-Smith, P. C., and Lewin, W. (1969). Cortical blindness and the functions of the non-geniculate fibres of the optic tracts. *J. Neurol. Neurosurg. Psychiat.* **32**, 259–64.

Broadbent, D. E. and Weiskrantz, L. (ed.) (1982). *The neuropsychology of cognitive function.* The Royal Society, London.

Brodmann, K. (1909). *Principien dargestellt auf Grund des Zellenbaues.* J. A. Barth, Leipzig.

Campion, J., Latto, R., and Smith, Y. M. (1983). Is blindsight an effect of scattered light, spared cortex, and near-threshold vision? *Beh. Brain Sci.* **6**, 423–48.

Churchland, P. S. (1980). A perspective on mind–brain research. *J. Phil.* **77**, 185–207.

—— (1983). Consciousness: the transmutation of a concept. *Pacific Phil. Quart.* **64**, 80–95.

Claparède, E. (1911). Récognition et moïté. *Arch. Psychol. Geneva* **11**, 79–90.

Cowey, A. (1961). *Perimetry in monkeys.* Ph.D. thesis, Univ. of Cambridge.

—— (1963). The basis of a method of perimetry with monkeys. *Q. Jl exp. Psychol.* **15**, 81–90.

—— (1967). Perimetric study of field defects in monkeys after cortical and retinal ablations. *Q. Jl exp. Psychol.* **19**, 232–45.

—— (1974). Atrophy of retinal ganlion cells after removal of striate cortex in a rhesus monkey. *Perception* **3**, 257–60.

—— (1985). Aspects of cortical organization related to selective attention and selective impairments of visual perception. In *Attention and Performance*, 11 (ed. M. I. Posner and O. S. M. Marin), pp. 41–62. Lawrence Erlbaum, Hillsdale, N.J.

—— and Perry, V. H. (1985). Cells and pathways for blindsight. Paper presented at European Brain and Behaviour Society Meeting, Oxford.

—— and Weiskrantz, L. (1963). A perimetric study of visual field defects in monkeys. *Q. Jl exp. Psychol.* **15**, 91–115.

Damasio, A., Lima, A., and Damasio, H. (1975). Nervous function after right hemispherectomy. *Neurol.* **25**, 89–93.

Darwin, C. (1871). *The descent of Man*. John Murray, London. (Page citations from 1894 edn.)

De Monasterio, F. M. (1978). Properties of ganglion cells with atypical receptive field organization in retina of macaques. *J. Neurophysiol.* **41**, 1435–49.

Denny-Brown, D. and Chambers, R. A. (1955). Visuo-motor function in the cerebral cortex. *J. nerv. ment. Dis.* **121**, 288–9.

Dichgans, J., Held, R., and Young, L. (1972). Moving visual scenes influence the apparent direction of gravity. *Science* **178**, 1217–19.

Dixon, N. F. (1971). *Subliminal perception. The nature of a controversy*. McGraw-Hill, London.

Efron, R. (1968). What is perception? *Boston studies in the philosophy of science*, pp. 137–73. Humanities Press, New York.

Fehrer, E. and Biederman, I. (1967). A comparison of reaction time and verbal report in the detection of masked stimuli. *J. exp. Psychol.* **64**, 126–30.

Ferrier, D. (1886). *The functions of the brain* (2nd ed.). Smith, Elder and Co., London.

Fries, W. (1981). The projection from the lateral geniculate nucleus to the prestriate cortex of the macaque monkey. *Proc. Roy. Soc. B*, **213**, 73–80.

Gaffan, D. (1974). Recognition impaired and association intact in the memory of monkeys after transection of the fornix. *J. comp. physiol. Psychol.* **86**, 1100–9.

Goldberg, M. E. and Wurtz, R. H. (1972). Activity of superior colliculus in behaving monkey. I. Visual reception fields of single neurons. *J. Neurophysiol.* **35**, 542–59.

Goldstein, K. and Gelb, A. (1918). Psychologische Analysen hirnpathologischer Fälle auf Grund von Untersuchungen Hirnverletzter. I. Abhandlung. Zur Psychologie des optischen Warnehmungs und Erkennungsvorganges. *Zeig. fur gesamte Neurol. u. Psychiat.* **41**, 1–142.

Goodale, M. A. (1973). Corticotectal and intertectal modulation of visual responses in the rat's superior colliculus. *Exp. Brain Res.* **17**, 75–86.

—— (1980). Visuomotor deficits in patients with progressive supranuclear palsy. Paper delivered to the International Neuropsychological Society, San Francisco.

—— (1981). Neural mechanisms of visual orientation in rodents: targets vs places. In *Spatially oriented behavior* (ed. A. Hein and M. Jeannerod). Springer-Verlag, Berlin.

—— and Lister, T. M. (1974). Attention to novel stimuli in rats with lesions of the superior colliculus. *Brain Res.* **66**, 361–2.

—— and Milner, A. D. (1982). Fractionating orientation behavior in the rodent: the role of the superior colliculus. In *The analysis of visual behavior* (ed. D. Ingle, M. A. Goodale, and R. Mansfield). M.I.T. Press, Cambridge, Mass.

—— and Murison, R. C. C. (1975). The effect of lesions of the superior colliculus on locomotor orientation and the orienting reflex in the rat. *Brain Res.* **88**, 243–61.

——, Foreman, N. P., and Milner, A. D. (1978). Visual orientation in the rat: a dissociation of deficits following cortical and collicular lesions. *Exp. Brain Res.* **31**, 445–57.

Gregory, R. L. (1972). Cognitive contours. *Nature, Lond.* **238**, 51–52.

Haymaker, W. (1953). *The founders of neurology*. Charles C. Thomas, Springfield.

Heywood, C. A. and Cowey, A. (1985). A comparison of the effects of superior collicular ablation in infant and adult rats. *Exp. Brain Res.* **59**, 302–12.

Heywood, S. and Ratcliff, G. (1976). Long-term oculomotor consequences of unilateral colliculectomy in man. In *Basic mechanisms of ocular motility and their clinical implications* (ed. G. Lennerstrand and P. Bach-y-Rita), pp. 561–4. Pergamon Press, Oxford.

Holmes, G. (1918). Disturbances of vision by cerebral lesions. *Brit. J. Ophthal.* **2**, 353–84.

—— (1945). The organization of the visual cortex in man. (Ferrier Lecture). *Proc. Roy. Soc. B,* **132**, 348–61.

—— and Lister, W. T. (1916). Disturbances of vision from cerebral lesions, with special reference to the cortical representation of macula. *Brain* **39**, 34–73.

Humphrey, N. K. (1970). What the frog's eye tells the monkey's brain. *Brain, Beh. Evol.* **3**, 324–37.

—— (1972). Seeing and nothingness. *New Scientist* **53**, 682–4.

—— (1974). Vision in a monkey without striate cortex: a case study. *Perception* **3**, 241–55.

—— and Weiskrantz, L. (1967). Vision in monkeys after removal of the striate cortex. *Nature, Lond.* **215**, 595–7.

Ingle, D. (1967). Two visual mechanisms underlying the behavior of fish. *Psychol. Forsch.* **31**, 44–51.

James, Wm. (1890). *Principles of psychology.* London: Macmillan and Co.

—— (1892). *Text-book of psychology.* Macmillan and Co., London.

Klüver, H. (1927). Visual disturbances after cerebral lesions. *Psychol. Bull.* **24**, 316–58.

—— (1942). Functional significance of the geniculo-striate system. *Biol. Sympos.* **7**, 253–99.

Koerner, F. and Teuber, H-L. (1973). Visual field defects after missile injuries to the geniculo-striate pathway in man. *Exp. Brain Res.* **18**, 88–112.

Kolb, B. and Whishaw, I. Q. (1985). *Fundamentals of human neuropsychology.* W. H. Freeman, New York.

Kuhn, T. S. (1962). *The structure of scientific revolutions.* Univ. Chicago Press, Chicago.

Lee, W. (1971). *Decision theory and human behavior.* Wiley, New York.

Lepore, F., Cardu, B., Rasmussen, T., and Malmo, R. B. (1975). Rod and cone sensitivity in destriate monkeys. *Brain Res.* **93**, 203–21.

Loeb, J. (1886). Beiträge zur Physiologie des Grosshirns. *Pflüger's Archiv.* **39**, 265–346.

Luciani, L. (1884). On the sensorial localisations in the cortex cerebri. *Brain* **7**, 145–60.

MacCurdy, J. T. (1928). *Common principles in psychology and physiology.* Cambridge Univ. Press, Cambridge.

Malmo, R. B. (1966). Effects of striate cortex ablation on intensity discrimination and spectral intensity distribution in the rhesus monkey. *Neuropsychologia* **4**, 9–26.

Marcel, A. J. (1983a). Conscious and unconscious perception: experiments on visual masking and word recognition. *Cog. Psychol.* **15**, 197–237.

—— (1983b). Conscious and unconscious perception: an approach to the relations between phenomenal experience and perceptual processes. *Cog. Psychol.* **15**, 238–300.

Marie, P. and Chatelin, C. (1915). Les troubles visuels dus aux lésions des voies optiques intra-cérébrales et de la sphère visuelle corticale dans les blessures du crâne par coup de feu. *Rev. neurol.* **28**, 882–925.

Marquis, D. G. (1935). Phylogenetic interpretation of the functions of the visual cortex. *Arch. Neurol. Psychiat.* **33**, 807–15.
—— and Hilgard, E. R. (1937). Conditioned responses to light in monkeys after removal of the occipital lobes. *Brain* **60**, 1–12.
Marzi, C. A., Tassinari, G., Lutzemberger, L., and Aglioti, S. (1985). Spatial summation across the visual vertical meridian in normal and hemianopic patients. Paper delivered at meeting of European Brain and Behaviour Society, Oxford.
Miller, M., Pasik, P., and Pasik, T. (1980). Extrageniculate vision in the monkey. VII. Contrast sensitivity functions. *J. Neurophysiol.* **43**, 1510–26.
Milner, A. D., Goodale, M. A., and Morton, M. C. (1979). Visual sampling after lesions of the superior colliculus in rats. *J. comp. physiol. Psychol.* **93**, 1015–23.
——, Lines, C. R., and Migdal, B. (1984). Visual orientation and detection following lesions of the superior colliculus in rats. *Exp. Brain Res.* **56**, 106–114.
Mohler, C. W. and Wurtz, R. H. (1977). Role of striate cortex and superior colliculus in visual guidance of saccadic eye movements in monkeys. *J. Neurophysiol.* **40**, 74–94.
Monakow, C. von (1914). *Die Lokalization im Grosshirn*. Bergmann, Weisbaden.
Morgan, C. Lloyd (1890). *Animal life and intelligence*. Edward Arnold, London.
Nakamura, R. K. and Mishkin, M. (1980). Blindness in monkeys following non-visual cortical lesions. *Brain Res.* **188**, 572–7.
Natsoulas, T. (1982). Conscious perception and the paradox of 'blind-sight'. In *Aspects of consciousness* vol. 3 (ed. G. Underwood). Academic Press, New York.
Paillard, J., Michel, F., and Stelmach, G. (1983). Localization without content: a tactile analogue of 'blind sight'. *Arch. Neurol.* **40**, 548–51.
Pasik, P. and Pasik, T. (1964). Oculomotor function in monkeys with lesions of the cerebrum and the superior colliculi. In *The Oculomotor System* (ed. M. B. Bender), pp. 40–80. Hoeber, New York.
Pasik, T. and Pasik, P. (1971). The visual world of monkeys deprived of striate cortex: effective stimulus parameters and the importance of the accessory optic system. In *Visual processes in vertebrates* (ed. T. Shipley and J. E. Dowling), Vision Research Supplement no. 3, pp. 419–35. Pergamon Press, Oxford.
—— —— (1980). Extrageniculostriate vision in primates. In *Neuro-ophthalmology* vol. 1 (ed. S. Lessell and J. T. W. van Dalen), pp. 95–119. Elsevier North-Holland, Amsterdam.
Perenin, M. T. (1978). Visual function within the hemianopic field following early cerebral hemidecortication in man. II. Pattern discrimination. *Neuropsychologia* **16**, 696–708.
——, Girard-Madoux, Ph., and Jeannerod, M. (1985). From completion to residual vision in hemianopic patients. Paper delivered at meeting of European Brain and Behaviour Society, Oxford.
—— and Jeannerod, M. (1975). Residual vision in cortically blind hemifields. *Neuropsychologia* **13**, 1–7.
—— —— (1978). Visual function within the hemianopic field following early cerebral hemidecortication in man. I. Spatial localization. *Neuropsychologia* **16**, 1–13.
—— —— (1983). Are extrageniculostriate pathways nonfunctional in man? *Beh. Brain Sci.* **6**, 458–9.
——, Ruel, J., and Hécaen, H. (1980). Residual visual capacities in a case of cortical blindness. *Cortex* **16**, 605–12.
Perry, V. H. and Cowey, A. (1984). Retinal ganglion cells that project to the superior collicular and pretectum in the macaque monkey. *Neuroscience* **12**(4), 1125–37.

——, Oehler, R., and Cowey, A. (1984). Retinal galgion cells that project to the dorsal lateral geniculate nucleus in the macaque monkey. *Neuroscience* **12**(4), 1101-23.

Pizzamiglio, L., Antonucci, G., and Francia, A. (1984). Response of the cortically blind hemifields to a moving visual scene. *Cortex* **20**, 89-99.

Poggio, G. F. (1968). Central neural mechanisms in vision. In *Medical physiology* (ed. V. B. Mountcastle). Mosby, St. Louis.

Pöppel, E. and Richards, W. (1974). Light sensitivity in cortical scotomata contralateral to small islands of blindness. *Exp. Brain Res.* **21**, 125-30.

——, Held, R., and Frost, D. (1973). Residual visual function after brain wounds involving the central visual pathways in man. *Nature, Lond.* **243**, 295-6.

Poppelreuter, W. (1917). *Die psychischen Schädigungen durch Kopfschuss im Kriege 1914-16; die Störungen der niederen und höheren Sehleistungen durch Verletzungen des Okzipitalhirns*, Vol. I. Voss, Leipzig.

Posner, M. I., Cohen, Y., and Rafal, R. D. (1982). Neural systems control of spatial orienting. In *Neuropsychology of cognitive function* (ed. D. E. Broadbent and L. Weiskrantz), pp. 187-98. The Royal Society, London.

Pötzl, O. and Redlich, E. (1911). Demonstration eines Falles von bilateraler Affektion beider Occipitallappen. *Wiener Klinische Wochenschrift* **24**, 517-18.

Richards, W. (1973). Visual processing in scotomata. *Exp. Brain Res.* **17**, 333-47.

Riddoch, G. (1917). Dissociation of visual perceptions due to occipital injuries, with especial reference to appreciation of movement. *Brain* **40**, 15-57.

Ruddock, K. H. and Waterfield, V. A. (1978). Selective loss of function associated with a central visual defect. *Neurosci. Letters* **8**, 93-8.

Sanders, M. D., Warrington, E. K., Marshall, J., and Weiskrantz, L. (1974). 'Blindsight': vision in a field defect. *Lancet*, April 20, 707-8.

Schilder, P., Pasik, P., and Pasik, T. (1972). Extrageniculate vision in the monkey. III. Circle vs triangle and 'red vs green' discrimination. *Exp. Brain Res.* **14**, 436-48.

——, Pasik, T., and Pasik, P. (1971). Extrageniculate vision in the monkey. II. Demonstration of brightness discrimination. *Brain Res.* **32**, 383-98.

Schiller, P. H. and Koerner, F. (1971). Discharge characteristics of single units in superior colliculus of the alert rhesus monkey. *J. Neurophysiol.* **34**, 920-36.

—— and Malpeli, J. G. (1977). Properties and tectal projections of monkey ganglion cells. *J. Neurophysiol.* **40**, 428-45.

Schneider, G. E. (1967). Contrasting visuomotor functions of tectum and cortex in the golden hamster. *Psychol. Forsch.* **31**, 52-62.

Searle, J. R. (1979). The intentionality of intention and action. *Inquiry* **22**, 253-80.

Singer, W., Zihl, J., and Pöppel, E. (1977). Subcortical control of visual thresholds in humans: evidence for modality specific and retinotopically organized mechanisms of selective attention. *Exp. Brain Res.* **29**, 173-90.

Sprague, J. M. (1966). Interaction of cortex and superior colliculus in mediation of visually guided behavior in the cat. *Science* **153**, 1544-7.

Stevens, S. S. (1961). The psychophysics of sensory function. In *Sensory communication* (ed. W. A. Rosenblith), pp. 1-33. Wiley, New York.

Stoerig, P., Hübner, M., and Pöppel, E. (1985). Signal detection analysis of residual vision in a field defect due to a post-geniculate lesion. *Neuropsychologia* **23**, 589-99.

ter Braak, J. W., Schenk, V. W. D., and van Vliet, A. G. M. (1971). Visual reactions in a case of long-standing cortical blindness. *J. Neurol. Neurosurg. Psychiat.* **34**, 140-47.

Teuber, H-L. (1965). Alterations of perception after brain injury. In *Study week on brain and conscious experience*, p. 274. Pontifical Academy of Sciences, Vatican City.

——, Battersby, W. S., and Bender, M. B. (1960). *Visual field defects after penetrating missle wounds of the brain.* Harvard Univ. Press, Cambridge, Mass.

Torjussen, T. (1976). Residual function in cortically blind hemifields. *Scand. J. Psychol.* **17**, 320–2.

—— (1978). Visual processing in cortically blind hemifields. *Neuropsychologia* **16**, 15–21.

Travel, D. and Damasio, A. R. (1985). Knowledge without awareness: an autonomic index of facial recognition by prosopagnosics. *Science* **228**, 1453–5.

Trevarthen, C. B. (1968). Two mechanisms of vision in primates. *Psychol. Forsch.* **31**, 299–337.

Turvey, M. T. (1973). On peripheral and central processes in vision: inferences from an information-processing analysis of masking with patterned stimuli. *Psychol. Rev.* **80**, 1–52.

Underwood, G. (1983). Verbal reports and visual awareness. *Beh. Brain Sci.* **6**, 463–4.

Van Buren, K. M. (1963). *The retinal ganglion cell layer.* Charles Thomas, Illinois.

Warrington, E. K. (1962). The completion of visual forms across hemianopic field defects. *J. Neurol. Neurosurg. Psychiat.* **25**, 208–17.

—— (1985). Agnosia: the impairment of object recognition. In *Handbook of clinical neurology*, **1** (45) (ed. J. A. M. Frederiks) pp. 333–49. Elsevier Science, Amsterdam.

—— and Taylor, A. M. (1973). The contribution of the right parietal lobe to object recognition. *Cortex* **9**, 152–64.

—— and Weiskrantz, L. (1968). New method of testing long-term retention with special reference to amnesic patients. *Nature, Lond.* **217**, 972–4.

—— —— (1982). Amnesia: a disconnection syndrome? *Neuropsychologia* **20**, 233–48.

Weiskrantz, L. (1961). Encephalisation and the scotoma. In *Current problems in animal behaviour* (eds. W. H. Thorpe and O. L. Zangwill), pp. 30–58. Cambridge Univ. Press, Cambridge.

—— (1963). Contour discrimination in a young monkey with striate cortex ablation. *Neuropsychologia* **1**, 145–64.

—— (1972). Behavioural analysis of the monkey's visual nervous system. (Review Lecture). *Proc. Roy. Soc. B*, **182**, 427–55.

—— (1977). Trying to bridge some neuropsychological gaps between monkey and man. *Br. J. Psychol.* **68**, 431–3.

—— (1978). Some aspects of visual capacity in monkeys and man following striate cortex lesions. *Arch. Ital. Biol.* **116**, 318–23.

—— (1980). Varieties of residual experience. *Q. Jl exp. Psychol.* **32**, 365–86.

—— (1983). Evidence and scotomata. *Beh. Brain Sci.* **6**, 464–7.

—— (1985a). On issues and theories of the human amnesic syndrome. In *Memory systems of the brain: animal and human cognitive processes* (eds. N. M. Weinberger, J. L. McGaugh, and G. Lynch), pp. 380–415. Guilford Press, New York.

—— (1985b). Introduction: categorization, cleverness, and consciousness. In *Animal intelligence* (ed. L. Weiskrantz), pp. 3–19. Oxford Univ. Press, Oxford.

—— (in press). Some contributions of neuropsychology of vision and memory to the problem of consciousness. In *Status of consciousness in contemporary science* (ed. E. Bisiach and A. J. Marcel).

—— and Cowey, A. (1963). Striate cortex lesions and visual acuity of the rhesus monkey. *J. comp. physiol. Psychol.* **56**, 225–31.

—— —— (1967). A comparison of the effects of striate cortex and retinal lesions on visual acuity in the monkey. *Science* **155**, 104–6.

—— —— (1970). Filling in the scotoma: a study of residual vision after striate cortex lesions in monkeys. In *Progress in physiological psychology*, vol. 3, (eds. E. Stellar and J. M. Sprague), pp. 237–60. Academic Press, New York.

—— ——, and Passingham, C. (1977). Spatial responses to brief stimuli by monkeys with striate cortex ablations. *Brain* **100**, 655–70.

—— and Warrington, E. K. (in press). A follow-up study of 'form' vision in a scotoma with residual vision. *Brain*.

—— ——, Sanders, M. D., and Marshall, J. (1974). Visual capacity in the hemianopic field following a restricted occipital ablation. *Brain* **97**, 709–28.

Werth, R. (1983). 'Blindsight': some conceptual considerations. *Beh. Brain Sci.* **6**, 467–8.

Wilbrand, H. and Saenger, A. (1918). *Die Verletzungen der Sehbahnen des Gehirns mit besonderer Berücksichtigung der Kriegsverletzungen.* Bergmann, Wiesbaden.

Wilson, M. E. (1968). The detection of light scattered from stimuli in impaired regions of the visual field. *J. Neurol. Neurosurg. Psychiat.* **31**, 509–13.

Yoshida, K. and Benevento, L. A. (1981). The projection from the dorsal geniculate nucleus of the thalamus to extrastriate visual association cortex in the macaque monkey. *Neurosci. Letters* **22**, 103–8.

Zihl, J. (1980). 'Blindsight': improvement of visually guided eye movements by systematic practice in patients with cerebral blindness. *Neuropsychologia* **18**, 71–7.

—— (1981). Recovery of visual functions in patients with cerebral blindness. *Exp. Brain Res.* **44**, 159–69.

—— and von Cramon, D. (1979). Restitution of visual function in patients with cerebral blindness. *J. Neurol. Neurosurg. Psychiat.* **42**, 312–22.

—— —— (1980). Registration of light stimuli in the cortically blind hemifield and its effect on localization. *Beh. Brain Res.* **1**, 287–98.

—— —— (1985). Visual field recovery from scotoma in patients with postgeniculate damage: a review of 55 cases. *Brain* **108**, 335–65.

—— ——, and Mai, N. (1983). Selective disturbance of movement vision after bilateral brain damage. *Brain* **106**, 313–40.

—— and Werth, R. (1984a). Contributions to the study of 'blindsight' — I. Can stray light account for saccadic localization in patients with postgeniculate field defects? *Neuropsychologia* **22**, 1–11.

—— —— (1984b). Contributions to the study of 'blindsight' — II. The role of specific practice for saccadic localization in patients with postgeniculate visual field defects. *Neuropsychologia* **22**, 13–22.

——, Tretter, F., and Singer, W. (1980). Phasic electrodermal responses after visual stimulation in the cortically blind hemifield. *Beh. Brain Res.* **1**, 197–203.

Author Index

183

Subject Index